Ninja Foodi Grill

Cookbook for Beginners

550 Easy, Quick and Delicious Recipes for Indoor Grilling and Air Frying Perfection

Table of Contents

Chapter 1: The Ninja Foodi Grill

The Benefits of The Ninja Foodi Grill
How to Use the Ninja Foodi Grill?
Tricks to Make Cooking Mistakes Avoid
Care & Cleaning Your Ninja Foodi Grill

Chapter 2: Breakfast

Crispy Garlic Potatoes
Spicy Sausage & Mushroom Casserole
Breakfast Omelette
Eggs & Avocado
French Toast
Hash Browns
Breakfast Potatoes
Breakfast Casserole
Breakfast Burrito
Ham & Cheese Casserole
French Toast Sticks
Bacon
Breakfast Bell Peppers
Sausage Casserole
Roasted Breakfast Potatoes

Chapter 3: Chicken & Turkey

Basil and Garlic Chicken Legs
Alfredo Chicken Apples
Hearty Chicken Zucchini Kabobs
Fried Chicken
Moroccan Roast Chicken
Chicken Zucchini Kebabs
Delicious Maple Glazed Chicken
Fried Chicken Thighs
Chicken Chili and Beans
Sweet and Sour Chicken BBQ
Turkey Tomato Burgers
Lemon Roasted Chicken
Baked Coconut Chicken
Hot and Sassy BBQ Chicken
Grilled Orange Chicken

Chapter 4: Appetizers & Snacks

Delicious Grilled Honey Fruit Salad
Ninja Grill Hot Dogs
Broccoli Maple Grill
Grilled Eggplant
Pineapple with Cream Cheese Dip
Chicken Salad with Blueberry Vinaigrette
Honey Glazed Bratwurst
Creamed Potato Corns
Fully Grilled Sweet Honey Carrot
Tarragon Asparagus
Grilled Butternut Squash
Complete Italian Squash
Lovely Seasonal Broccoli
Mammamia Banana Boats
Cob with Pepper Butter

Chapter 5: Meat

Sausage & Pepper
Roast Beef with Garlic
Ranch Pork Chops
Steak Kebab
Cuban Pork Chops
Grilled Steak & Potatoes
Rib Eye Steak with Onions & Peppers
Tenderloin Steak with Bacon
Grilled Pork Chops
Paprika Pork Chops
Coffee Rib-eye
Roast Beef & Grilled Potatoes
Cheeseburger
Grilled Herbed Steak
Steak with Asparagus

Chapter 6: Vegetarian and Vegan

Delicious Cajun Eggplant
Cool Rosemary Potatoes
Olive and Spinach Crispies
Definitive Air Brussels
Mustard Dredged Veggie Delight
Zucchini and Egg Delight
Premium Broccoli and Garlic Meal

Charred up Shishito Pepper
The Creamy Potato Meal
Corny Creamy Potatoes
Epic Asparagus
Delicious Broccoli and Arugula
Exciting Granola Muffins
Corn and Mayo
Fruit Packed Lime Salad

Chapter 7: Fish and Seafood

Spanish Shrimp
Mustard Crispy Cod
Mesmerizing Parmesan Fish
Lemon Garlic Shrimp
Tuna Patties
Roast BBQ Shrimp
Crispy Crabby Patties
Tuna Patties
Salt and Pepper Shrimp
Spicy Grilled Shrimps
Buttery Spiced Grilled Salmon
Teriyaki Coho Glazed Salmon
Simple Grilled Swordfish
Coconut Shrimp

Chapter 8: Desserts, Bread & Rolls

A Fruit Salad to Die For
French Toast Bites
Lovely Rum Sundae
Fiery Cajun Eggplant Dish
Granola Flavored Healthy Muffin
Cinnamon Sugar Roasted Chickpeas
Marshmallow Banana Boat
Smoked Apple Crumble
Sweet Cream Cheese Wontons
Tuna Stuffed Potatoes
Cinnamon Fried Bananas
Bruschetta Portobello Mushrooms
Marshmallow Banana Boat
Baked Apple
Rummy Pineapple Sunday
Cherry-Choco Bars

Chapter 1: The Ninja Foodi Grill

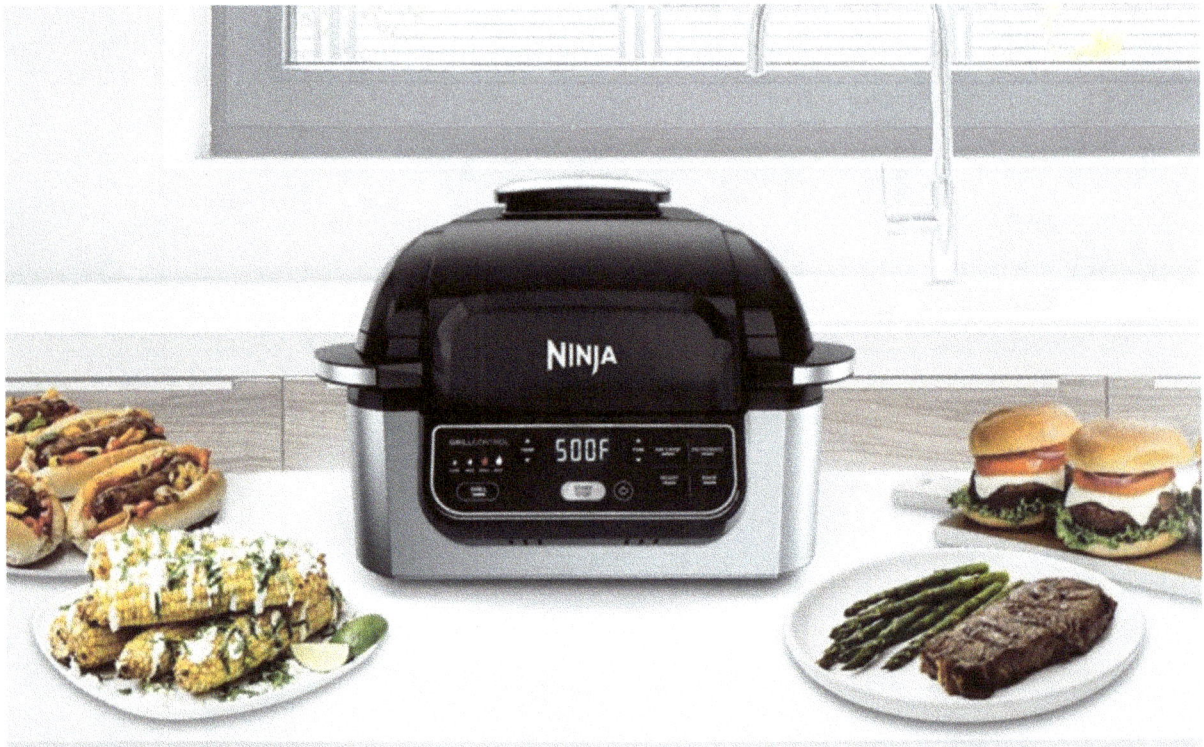

• Ninja Foodi Grill is nothing but convenience for those who love to enjoy nicely grilled food but too busy to set up an outdoor grill. It has brought innovation right at our fingertips by bringing all the necessary cooking in a digital one-touch device. It is simple to manage and control. And what makes the Ninja foodi grill apart from other electric grills is the diversity of options it provides for cooking all in a single pot. The ceramic coated interior and accessories make grilling an effortless experience. The Ninja Foodi grill is an electric grill, air fryer, convection oven, oven toaster, and dehydrator all rolled into one. This cookbook puts the idea of electric grill into perspective by discussing the basics of using the Ninja Foodi Grill. The company has launched the appliance with only one aim that is to provide convenient grilling for all. Try the flavorsome grilling recipes in your Ninja Food grills and experience good taste with amazing aroma, all with little efforts and lesser time.

•

The Benefits of The Ninja Foodi Grill

• Whether it is a trend or the general convenience of it, more people are appreciating smaller and more portable indoor cookers due to a number of benefits from owning one.

- Easy to clean and operate – Indoor grills are plug and play appliances making them user-friendly to a wider demographic. The cooking components are coated with a non-stick ceramic material that can be effortlessly taken apart and cleaned using a standard dishwasher.

- Smokeless – This is probably one of the best things about indoor electric grills. People who do not have any access to open areas can still enjoy grilling since it does not produce smoke like standard grillers.

- Multi-function – Most indoor cookers come with various functionalities giving you more value for your money. It can also eliminate the need to purchase other appliances and save you essential kitchen space.

- Compact – Electric grills are small enough to fit most kitchen counters and tables. It is also portable enough to be easily transported or moved around.

- Capable of high temperatures – A wide range of temperature settings let you cook a variety of foods from char-grilled vegetables to restaurant-level steaks. Unlike other tabletop cookers, the Ninja Grill will let you cook frozen foods without the need to defrost. It can also get as hot as 500 to 510 degrees Fahrenheit.

- Browns and crisps food – Indoor grills like the Ninja Foodi use the circulating hot air to cook the food thoroughly. This creates delectable flavors through a browning process called the Maillard reaction. Similar to convection ovens and toasters, the Ninja Foodi is excellent at making food crunchy when you need it to be.

- Grill marks - Like traditional outdoor grills, indoor grills can also give meat and other foods those appetizing grill marks. Although, the Ninja Foodi's grill marks are curved, unlike the typical straight markings you get from regular outdoor grills.

-

How to Use the Ninja Foodi Grill?

- When you are cooking for the first time with your Foodi grill, you must first wash the detachable cooking parts with warm soapy water to remove any oil and debris. Let them air dry and place them back inside once you are ready to cook. An easy-to-follow instruction guide comes with each unit, so make sure to go over it before cooking.

- Position your grill on a level and secure surface. Leave at least 6 inches of space around it, especially at the back where the air intake vent and air socket are located. Ensure that the splatter guard is installed whenever the grill is in use. This is a wire mesh that covers the heating element on the inside of the lid.

1. Grilling

• Plug your unit into an outlet and power on the grill.

• Use the grill grate over the cooking pot and choose the grill function. This has four default temperature settings of low at 400 degrees F, medium at 450 degrees F, high at 500 degrees F, and max at 510 degrees F.

• Set the time needed to cook. You may check the grilling cheat sheet that comes with your unit to guide you with the time and temperature settings. It is best to check the food regularly depending on the doneness you prefer and to avoid overcooking.

• Once the required settings are selected, press start and wait for the digital display to show 'add food'. The unit will start to preheat similar to an oven and will show the progress through the display. This step takes about 8 minutes.

• If you need to check the food or flip it, the timer will pause and resume once the lid is closed.

• The screen will show 'Done' once the timer and cooking have been completed. Power off the unit and unplug the device. Leave the hood open to let the unit cool faster.

2. Roasting

• Remove the grill grates and use the cooking pot that comes with the unit. You may also purchase their roasting rack for this purpose.

• Press the roast option and set the timer between 1 to 4 hours depending on the recipe requirements. The Foodi will preheat for 3 minutes regardless of the time you have set.

• Once ready, place the meat directly on the roasting pot or rack.

• Check occasionally for doneness. A meat thermometer is another useful tool to get your meats perfectly cooked.

3. Bake

• Remove the grates and use the cooking pot.

• Choose the bake setting and set your preferred temperature and time. Preheating will take about 3 minutes.

- Once done with preheating, you may put the ingredients directly on the cooking pot, or you may use your regular baking tray. An 8-inch baking tray can fit inside as well as similar-sized oven-safe containers.

4. Air crisping

- Put the crisper basket in and close the lid.

- Press the air crisp option then the start button. The default temperature is set at 390° F and will preheat at about 3 minutes. You can adjust the temperature and time by pressing the buttons beside these options.

- If you do not need to preheat, just press the air crisp button a second time and the display will show you the 'add food' message.

- Put the food inside and shake or turn every 10 minutes. Use oven mitts or tongs with silicone when doing this.

5. Dehydrating

- Place the first layer of food directly on the cooking pot.

- Add the crisper basket and add one more layer.

- Choose the dehydrate setting and set the timer between 7 to 10 hours.

- You may check the progress from time to time.

6.Cooking frozen foods

- Choose the medium heat, which is 450° F using the grill option. You may also use the air crisp option if you are cooking fries, vegetables, and other frozen foods.

- Set the time needed for your recipe. Add a few minutes to compensate for the thawing.

- Flip or shake after a few minutes to cook the food evenly.

Tricks to Make Cooking Mistakes Avoid

- There are plenty of things to remember, and many common errors to prevent to achieve a perfect Ninja Foodi grill steak. As a beginner, understanding what these grilling errors are, and how to avoid them, is critical. This way, you're on the right track to becoming a grilling pro in no time!

- Here are the most common grilling errors starters can avoid:

1. Uses bad resources

- Some of the most common myths about the Ninja Foodi grill are that to achieve delicious and perfectly cooked grilled dishes; you need fancy, expensive tools, and equipment. Despite this, many grillers make the mistake of either using needless or bad instruments. Save your money: You only need a few simple yet reliable tools to get the job done like a long-lasting pair of tongs, a spatula, heat-resistant gloves, a food thermometer, and some clean towels. Often opt for arm and hand safety with the long-handled variety of the tongs and spatula.

2. Meat thermometer not used

- One of the most common Ninja Foodi grill errors is to forego the food thermometer, which often leads to a grilled dish that is either overcooked or undercooked. You don't want visitors to get or see raw or burnt food, so be sure to invest in a decent thermometer to make it easier to read the internal temperatures. Don't worry; you'll know when the food is ready by looking at it once you get the hang of grilling. Meanwhile, get a decent quality food thermometer for yourself.

3. Too much sauce too soon

- There are plenty of grillers making the mistake of slathering the meat with sauce while cooking on the grill of Ninja Foodi. Most glazes, marinades, and sauces contain sugar that easily burns out. Because of this, it will burn your steak on the outside but still raw on the inside. If you want to cook your food evenly, add the right amount of sauce at the end of the grilling process approximately 10 minutes before your food is ready.

4. No time taken to prepare

- Are you aware that every successful cook's rule number 1 is "mis en place," which means all in place? It ensures that everything should be prepare before beginning the cooking process accordingly. The same goes for grilling on Ninja Foodi. Most grillers make the mistake of preparing certain ingredients while on the grill; this contributes to burning or uneven cooking. It is of utmost importance that all of your ingredients are ready. Once you light up, your grill-meat should be thawed and marinated, fruits and vegetables should be diced, sliced or peeled, and sauces mixed.

5. Holding a dirty grill

- Probably the most common grilling error is holding a dirty grill. Not regularly cleaning your Ninja Foodi grill is not only unhygienic but also increases the risk of hazards to your safety. Grease quickly builds up in your grill after just a few uses, which is the number one cause of flare-ups. Also, food can stick more easily to dirty grates that could lead to uneven cooking. If you can to prevent hazards, clean your grill after every use.

Care & Cleaning Your Ninja Foodi Grill

- It might appear very tricky to thoroughly clean the Ninja Foodi Grill, but it is not complicated at all. You merely need to follow certain easy steps, and your device is ready to go for another round. It is recommended to thoroughly clean the Ninja Foodi Grill after every use. To clean the unit thoroughly and safely, follow the following guidelines:

  - Let the device cool down before cleaning.
  - Unplug the device from the power source.
  - For quick cooling, keep the hood of the device open.
  - The grill gate, splatter shield, crisper basket, cooking pot, cleaning brush, and the rest of the accessories are certified as DISHWASHER SAFE.
  - The thermometer is not dishwasher safe.
  - Rinse the accessories like splatter shield, grill gate, etc. for better cleaning results.
  - Use the cleaning brush included with the device for handwashing.
  - For cleaning baked-on cheese or sauces, utilize the other end of the cleaning brush for being used as a scrapper for effective hand washing.
  - Either towel-dry or air-dry all the components after hand washing.
  - DO NOT dip the main unit in any liquid, including water.
  - DO NOT use any rasping cleaners or tools.
  - NEVER use any sort of liquid cleaning solution near or on the thermometer.
  - Always use a cotton swab or compressed air to avoid any damage to the jack.

- In case of any grease or food residue left and stuck on the components of the Ninja Foodi Grill, follow the following cleaning steps thoroughly:

  1. If the residue is stuck on the splatter shield, grill gate, or any other accessory or part, soak it in warm soapy water solution before cleaning.

2. The splatter should be cleaned thoroughly after every use. For better cleansing, soak it in warm water overnight will assists efficiently in softening the stuck grease or sauces.

3. You can also deep clean the splatter shield by thoroughly immersing it in water and further boiling it for approximately 10 minutes.

4. **Moreover, you can then rinse it effectively with room temperature water and let it dry properly for better results.**

• For deep cleaning the thermometer, you can soak both the silicone grip and the stainless-steel tip in a container full of warm water. But, keep in mind that the jack or the cord **SHOULD NOT** be immersed or soaked in any solution, including water, as mentioned earlier. The thermometer holder of the Ninja Foodi Grill is clearly **HANDWASH** only.

Chapter 2: Breakfast

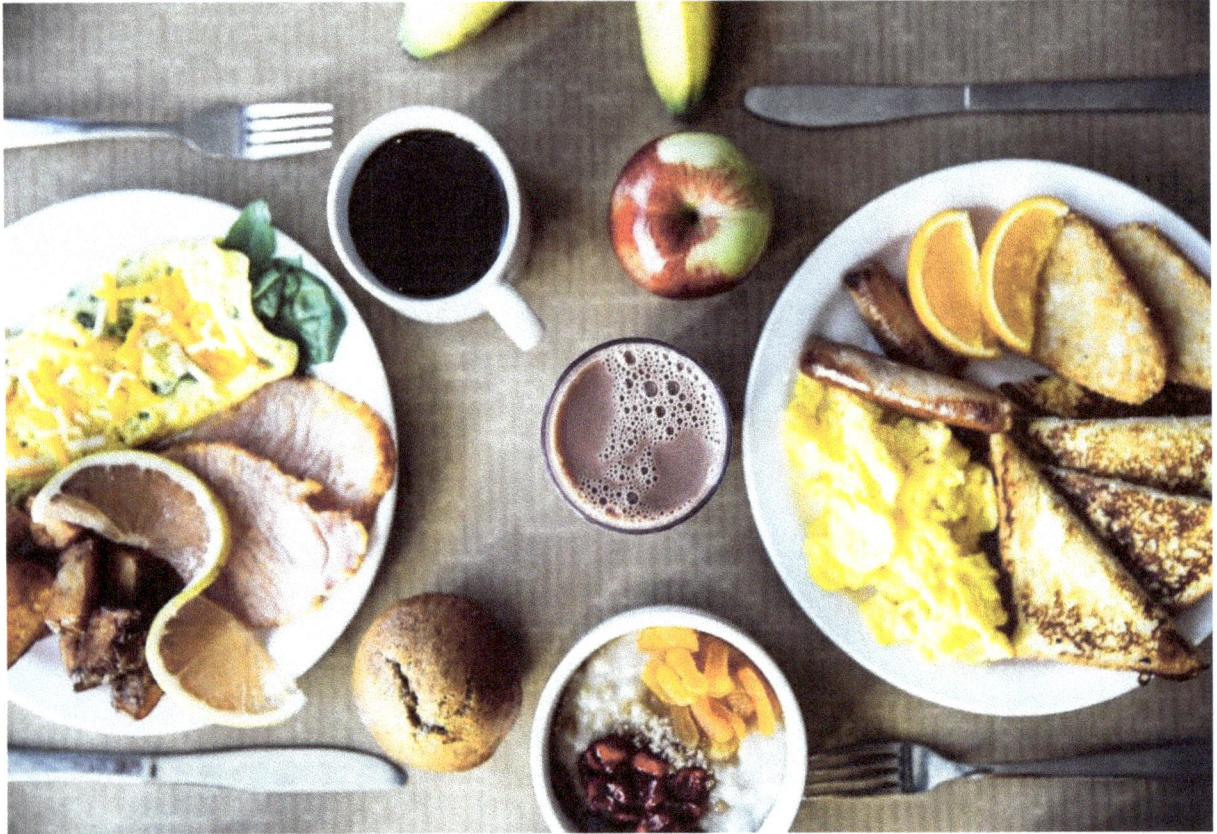

1.

Crispy Garlic Potatoes

Prep Time: 10 minutes

Cooking Time: 20 minutes

Serves: 8

Ingredients:

- 1 teaspoon garlic powder
- 1 1/2 lb. potatoes, diced
- 1 tablespoon avocado oil
- Salt and pepper to taste

Directions:

1. Toss the potatoes in oil.

2. Season with garlic powder, salt and pepper.

3. Add the air fryer basket to the Ninja Foodi Grill.

4. Select air crisp setting.

5. Cook at 400 degrees F for 20 minutes, tossing halfway through.

Serving Suggestions: Sprinkle with chopped turkey bacon crisps.

Preparation / Cooking Tips: You can also season the potatoes with paprika.

Spicy Sausage & Mushroom Casserole

Prep Time: 15 minutes

Cooking Time: 15 minutes

Serves: 6

Ingredients:

- 1 tablespoon olive oil
- 3/4 cup white onion, diced
- 1/4 cup cream of mushroom soup
- 3/4 cup cheddar cheese, shredded
- 5 mushrooms, sliced
- 1/2 lb. spicy ground sausage
- 8 eggs, beaten scrambled
- Garlic salt to taste

Directions:

1. In a pan over medium heat, pour the olive oil and cook onion, mushrooms and spicy ground sausage for 5 minutes.

2. Remove from heat and drain oil.

3. Pour eggs and sausage mixture into the Ninja Foodi Grill pot.

4. Season with garlic salt.

5. Spread mushroom soup on top.

6. Sprinkle with cheese.

7. Seal the pot.

8. Set to air crisp and cook at 390 degrees F for 5 minutes.

9. Stir and cook for another 5 minutes.

Serving Suggestions: Sprinkle with chopped chives before serving.

Preparation / Cooking Tips: You can use Alfredo pasta sauce if you don't have cream of mushroom soup.

Breakfast Omelette

Prep Time: 15 minutes

Cooking Time: 10 minutes

Serves: 6

Ingredients:

- 6 eggs
- 1 white onion, diced
- 2 slices ham, chopped and cooked
- 1 cup cheddar cheese, shredded
- 1 red bell pepper, diced
- 6 mushrooms, chopped
- Salt and pepper to taste

Directions:

1. Beat eggs in a bowl.

2. Stir in the rest of the ingredients.

3. Set your Ninja Foodi Grill to air crisp.

4. Pour the egg mixture into the pot.

5. Cook at 390 degrees F for 10 minutes, stirring halfway through.

Serving Suggestions: Serve with toasted garlic bread.

Preparation / Cooking Tips: You can also use turkey bacon to replace ham in this recipe.

Eggs & Avocado

Prep Time: 10 minutes

Cooking Time: 15 minutes

Serves: 2

Ingredients:

- 2 eggs
- 1 avocado, sliced in half and pitted
- Salt and pepper to taste
- Cheddar cheese, shredded

Directions:

1. Scoop out about a tablespoon of avocado flesh to make a hole.
2. Crack egg on top of the avocado.
3. Season with salt and pepper.
4. Sprinkle with cheese.
5. Air crisp at 390 degrees F for 12 to 15 minutes.

Serving Suggestions: Serve with salsa or hot sauce.

Preparation / Cooking Tips: Scoop out more avocado flesh to create a bigger hole for the egg.

French Toast

Prep Time: 15 minutes

Cooking Time: 10 minutes

Serves: 4

Ingredients:

- 6 eggs
- 1 cup milk
- Cooking spray
- 1 loaf French bread, sliced
- 1 teaspoon honey
- 1 cup heavy cream
- 1/2 cup sugar

- 1/2 cup butter

Directions:

2. Beat the eggs in a bowl.

3. Stir in milk, cream and honey.

4. Dip the bread slices into the mixture.

5. Add to the grill basket inside the Ninja Foodi Grill.

6. Spread some butter and sprinkle sugar on top of the bread slices.

7. Seal the pot and air crisp at 350 degrees F for 5 to 10 minutes.

Serving Suggestions: Serve with maple syrup.

Preparation / Cooking Tips: It's a good idea to use day-old bread for this recipe.

Hash Browns

Prep Time: 15 minutes

Cooking Time: 20 minutes

Serves: 4

Ingredients:

- 6 potatoes, grated
- 1 bell pepper, chopped
- 2 teaspoons olive oil
- 1 onion, chopped
- Salt and pepper to taste

Directions:

1. Toss the grated potatoes, onion and bell pepper separately in oil.

2. Season with salt and pepper.

3. Add potatoes to the Grill.

4. Air crisp at 400 degrees F for 10 minutes.

5. Shake and stir in onion and pepper.

6. Cook for another 10 minutes.

Serving Suggestions: Serve with side salad.

Preparation / Cooking Tips: Soak the potatoes in water for 30 minutes after grating. Dry completely with paper towels before cooking. Doing this technique results in a crispier hash brown.

Breakfast Potatoes

Prep Time: 15 minutes

Cooking Time: 55 minutes

Serves: 4

Ingredients:

- 4 potatoes
- 2 cups cheddar cheese, shredded
- 8 slices bacon, cooked crispy and chopped
- 1 1/4 cups sour cream
- 4 teaspoons butter

Directions:

1. Take out the grill gate and crisper basket.
2. Set Ninja Foodi Grill to bake.
3. Set it to 390 degrees F.
4. Preheat by selecting "start".
5. Add the potatoes inside.
6. Seal and cook for 45 minutes.
7. Let cool.
8. Make slices on top of the potatoes.
9. Create a small hole.
10. Top with butter and cheese.
11. Put the potatoes back to the pot.
12. Bake at 375 degrees F for 10 minutes.
13. Top with sour cream and bacon before serving.

Serving Suggestions: Garnish with chopped scallions.

Preparation / Cooking Tips: Preheat the Ninja Foodi Grill before putting back the potatoes back to the pot after cheese and butter have been added.

Breakfast Casserole

Prep Time: 15 minutes

Cooking Time: 15 minutes

Serves: 8

Ingredients:

- ¼ cup white onion, diced
- 1/2 cup Colby Jack cheese, shredded
- 8 eggs, beaten
- 1 green bell pepper, diced
- 1 lb. ground sausage, cooked
- Garlic salt to taste

Directions:

1. Add white onion, bell pepper and ground sausage to your Ninja Foodi Grill pot.
2. Spread cheese and then the eggs on top.
3. Season with garlic salt.
4. Set to air crisp and cook at 390 degrees F for 15 minutes.

Serving Suggestions: Garnish with chopped parsley.

Preparation / Cooking Tips: You can also place casserole in a small dish and put it inside the air fryer basket.

Breakfast Burrito

Prep Time: 15 minutes

Cooking Time: 30 minutes

Serves: 12

Ingredients:

- 1 teaspoon olive oil

- 1 lb. breakfast sausage
- 10 eggs, beaten
- 3 cups cheddar cheese, shredded
- 2 cups potatoes, diced
- Salt and pepper to taste
- 12 tortillas

Directions:

1. Pour olive oil into a pan over medium heat.
2. Cook potatoes and sausage for 7 to 10 minutes, stirring frequently.
3. Spread this mixture on the bottom of the Ninja Foodi Grill .
4. Season with salt and pepper.
5. Pour the eggs and cheese on top.
6. Select bake setting.
7. Cook at 325 degrees F for 20 minutes.
8. Top the tortilla with the cooked mixture and roll.
9. Sprinkle cheese on the top side.
10. Add the air fryer basket to the Ninja Foodi Grill.
11. Air crisp the burrito at 375 degrees F for 10 minutes.

Serving Suggestions: You can also serve this as snack.

Preparation / Cooking Tips: The burrito can be made ahead and frozen. Take it out of the freezer 30 minutes before cooking it.

Ham & Cheese Casserole

Prep Time: 15 minutes

Cooking Time: 20 minutes

Serves: 8

Ingredients:

- 1 lb. ham, chopped and cooked
- 1 red bell pepper, chopped

- 1 white onion, chopped
- 1 yellow bell pepper, chopped
- 2 cups Colby Jack cheese, shredded
- 8 eggs, beaten
- Salt and pepper to taste

Directions:

1. Line the air fryer basket with foil.
2. Spread ham on the bottom of the basket.
3. Top with the cheese, onion, bell peppers and eggs.
4. Sprinkle with salt and pepper.
5. Choose air crisp function.
6. Cook at 390 degrees F for 15 to 20 minutes.

Serving Suggestions: Sprinkle with grated Parmesan cheese before serving.

Preparation / Cooking Tips: You can also use cheddar cheese in place of Colby Jack cheese.

French Toast Sticks

Prep Time: 10 minutes

Cooking Time: 10 minutes

Serves: 12

Ingredients:

- 5 eggs
- 1 cup almond milk
- 1 teaspoon vanilla extract
- 1/4 cup sugar
- 4 tablespoons melted butter
- 4 bread slices, sliced into 12 sticks

Directions:

1. Beat the eggs in a bowl.
2. Stir in milk, sugar, vanilla and butter.

3. Dip the bread sticks into the mixture.

4. Add these to the air fryer basket and place inside the Ninja Foodi Grill.

5. Air crisp at 350 degrees F for 8 to 10 minutes.

Serving Suggestions: Sprinkle with cinnamon powder before serving.

Preparation / Cooking Tips: Prepare in advance and freeze for later use.

Bacon

Prep Time: 5 minutes

Cooking Time: 10 minutes

Serves: 3

Ingredients:

- 2 tablespoons water
- 6 slices bacon

Directions:

1. Pour water to the bottom of the Ninja Foodi Grill pot.

2. Place the grill rack inside.

3. Put the bacon slices on the grill rack.

4. Select air crisp function.

5. Cook at 350 degrees F for 5 minutes per side or until golden and crispy.

Serving Suggestions: Serve with bread and vegetables for a complete breakfast meal.

Preparation / Cooking Tips: Use turkey bacon if you want a breakfast dish that's lower in fat and cholesterol.

Breakfast Bell Peppers

Prep Time: 10 minutes

Cooking Time: 15 minutes

Serves: 2

Ingredients:

- 4 eggs, beaten

- 1 large bell pepper, sliced in half
- 1 teaspoon olive oil
- Salt and pepper to taste

Directions:

1. Brush the bell pepper halves with oil.
2. Pour eggs into the bell pepper.
3. Sprinkle with salt and pepper.
4. Place these in the air fryer basket.
5. Set the Ninja Foodi Grill to air crisp.
6. Cook at 390 degrees F for 15 minutes.

Serving Suggestions: Sprinkle with chopped parsley before serving.

Preparation / Cooking Tips: You can also crack the eggs into the bell peppers.

Sausage Casserole

Prep Time: 15 minutes

Cooking Time: 20 minutes

Serves: 4

Ingredients:

- 1 lb. hash browns
- 2 red bell peppers, chopped
- 1 white onion, chopped
- 4 eggs, beaten
- 1 lb. ground breakfast sausage, cooked
- Salt and pepper to taste

Directions:

1. Line the air fryer basket with foil.
2. Add hash browns at the bottom part.
3. Spread sausage, onion and bell peppers on top.
4. Air crisp at 355 degrees F for 10 minutes.

5. Pour eggs on top and cook for another 10 minutes.

6. Season with salt and pepper.

Serving Suggestions: Garnish with chopped herbs.

Preparation / Cooking Tips: You can also use turkey sausage for this recipe.

Roasted Breakfast Potatoes

Prep Time: 15 minutes

Cooking Time: 25 minutes

Serves: 4

Ingredients:

- 3 large potatoes, diced
- Garlic salt and pepper to taste
- 1 tablespoon butter
- 3 sprigs thyme
- 1 tablespoon olive oil
- 2 sprigs rosemary

Directions:

1. Add potatoes to the Ninja Foodi Grill pot.
2. Toss in olive oil and butter.
3. Season with garlic salt and pepper.
4. Top with the herb sprigs.
5. Seal the pot.
6. Set it to air crisp.
7. Cook at 375 degrees F for 25 minutes.

Serving Suggestions: Garnish with chopped parsley.

Preparation / Cooking Tips: Stir the potatoes halfway through to ensure even cooking.

8.

Chapter 3: Chicken & Turkey

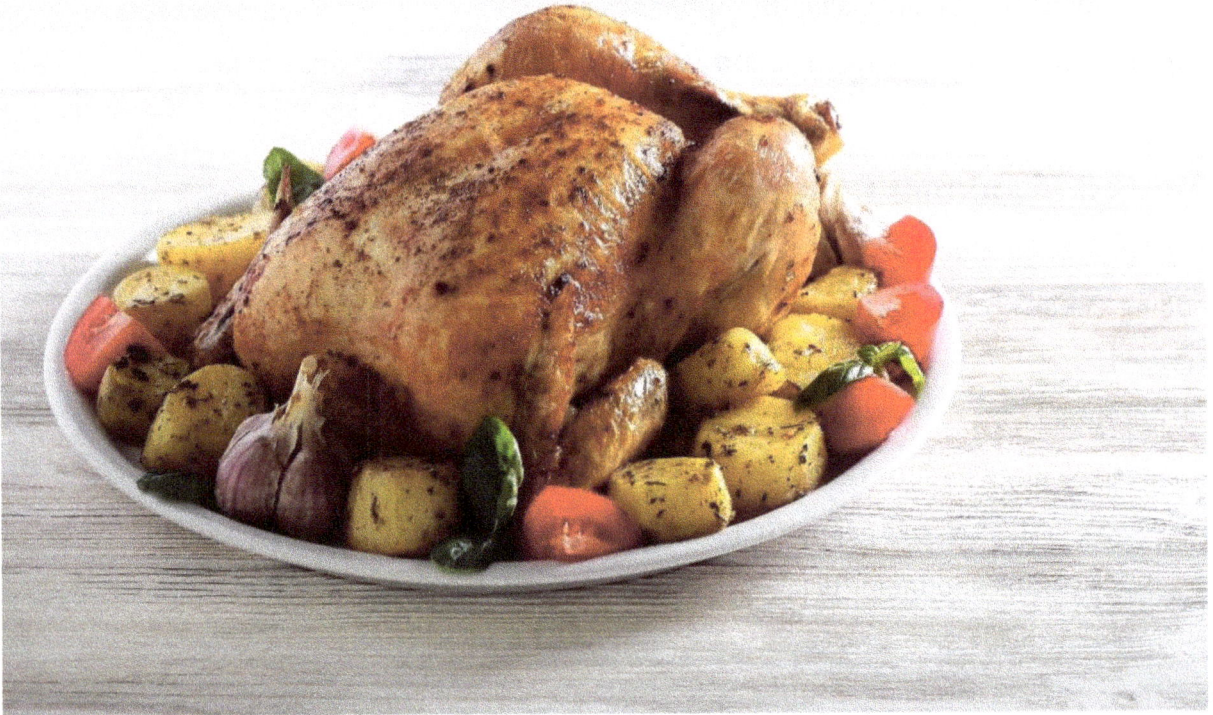

9.

Basil and Garlic Chicken Legs

Prep Time: 10 minutes

Cooking Time: 35 minutes

Serves: 4

Ingredients:

- 4 chicken legs
- 2 teaspoons garlic, minced
- 1 lemon, sliced
- 2 tablespoons olive oil
- 4 teaspoons basil, dried
- Pinch of pepper and salt

Directions:

1. Pre-heat Ninja Foodi by squeezing the "AIR CRISP" alternative and setting it to "350 Degrees F" and timer to 20 minutes
2. Coat chicken with oil using a brush and drizzle with rest of the ingredients
3. Transfer to Ninja Foodi Grill
4. Add lemon slices around the chicken legs
5. Close the Grill
6. Cook for 20 minutes
7. Serve and enjoy!

Nutrition:

Calories: 240, Fat: 18 g, Saturated Fat: 4 g, Carbohydrates: 3 g, Fiber: 2 g, Sodium: 1253 mg

Alfredo Chicken Apples

Prep Time: 5-10 minutes

Cooking Time: 20 minutes

Serves: 4

Ingredients:

- 1 large apple, wedged
- 4 teaspoon chicken seasoning
- 4 slices provolone cheese
- 1 tablespoon lemon juice
- ¼ cup blue cheese, crumbled
- 4 chicken breasts, halved
- ½ cup alfredo sauce

Directions:

1. Take a bowl and add chicken, season it well
2. Take another bowl and add in apple, lemon juice
3. Pre-heat Ninja Foodi by pressing the "GRILL" option and setting it to "MED" and timer to 20 minutes
4. Let it pre-heat until you hear a beep

5. Arrange chicken over Grill Grate, lock lid and cook for 8 minutes, flip and cook for 8 minutes more

6. Grill apple in the same manner for 2 minutes per side (making sure to remove chicken beforehand)

7. Serve chicken with pepper, apple, blue cheese, and alfredo sauce

8. Enjoy!

Nutrition:

Calories: 247, Fat: 19 g, Saturated Fat: 6 g, Carbohydrates: 29 g, Fiber: 6 g, Sodium: 853 mg, Protein: 14 g

Hearty Chicken Zucchini Kabobs

Prep Time: 10 minutes

Cooking Time: 15 minutes

Serves: 4

Ingredients:

- 1-pound chicken breast, boneless, skinless and cut into cubes of 2 inches
- ¼ cup extra-virgin olive oil
- 2 tablespoons oregano
- 2 tablespoons Greek yogurt, plain
- 4 lemons juice
- 1 red onion, quartered
- 1 zucchini, sliced
- 1 lemon zest
- ½ teaspoon ground black pepper
- 4 garlic cloves, minced
- 1 teaspoon of sea salt

Directions:

1. Take a mixing bowl, add the Greek yogurt, lemon juice, oregano, garlic, zest, salt, and pepper, combine them well

2. Add the chicken and coat well, refrigerate for 1-2 hours to marinate

3. Arrange the grill grate and close the lid

4. Pre-heat Ninja Foodi by pressing the "GRILL" option and setting it to "MED" and timer to 7 minutes

5. Take the skewers, thread the chicken, zucchini and red onion and thread alternatively

6. Let it pre-heat until you hear a beep

7. Arrange the skewers over the grill grate lock lid and cook until the timer reads zero

8. Baste the kebabs with a marinating mixture in between

9. Take out your when it reaches 165 degrees F

10. Serve warm and enjoy!

Nutrition:

Calories: 277, Fat: 15 g, Saturated Fat: 4 g, Carbohydrates: 10 g, Fiber: 2 g, Sodium: 146 mg

Fried Chicken

Prep Time: 10 minutes

Cooking Time: 25 minutes

Servings: 6

Ingredients:

- 6 chicken drumsticks, rinse and pat dry with a paper towel
  - tsp. ginger
- 1 tsp. onion powder
- 1 tsp. garlic powder
- 1 tsp. paprika
- 1 cup buttermilk
- ¼ cup brown sugar
- ½ cup breadcrumbs
- 1 cup all-purpose flour
- ½ tsp. pepper
- 1 tsp. salt

Directions:

1. Preheat the Ninja Foodi Grill using bake mode at 390 F.
2. Add breadcrumbs, spices, and flour into the zip-lock bag and mix well.
3. In a bowl, mix together chicken and buttermilk and let sit for 2 minutes.
4. Now put a single piece of chicken into the zip-lock bag and shake it until chicken is evenly coated with breadcrumb mixture. Do this same with remaining chicken pieces.
5. Spray coated chicken with cooking spray.
6. Place chicken into the bottom tray of the Ninja Foodi Grill and bake for 25 minutes.
7. Serve and enjoy.

Nutrition:

Calories 234, Fat 3.8 g, Carbohydrates 31.5 g, Sugar 8.7 g, Protein 17.6 g, Cholesterol 42 mg

Moroccan Roast Chicken

Prep Time: 5-10 minutes

Cooking Time: 22 minutes

Serves: 4

Ingredients:

- 3 tablespoons plain yogurt
- 4 skinless, boneless chicken thighs
- ½ teaspoon fresh flat-leaf parsley, chopped
- 2 teaspoons ground cumin
- 4 garlic cloves, chopped
- ½ teaspoon salt
- 2 teaspoons paprika
- ¼ teaspoon crushed red pepper flakes
- 1/3 cup olive oil

Directions:

1. Take your food processor and add garlic, yogurt, salt, oil and blend well

2. Take a mixing bowl and add chicken, red pepper flakes, paprika, cumin, parsley, garlic, and mix well

3. Let it marinate for 2-4 hours

4. Pre-heat Ninja Foodi by pressing the "ROAST" option and setting it to "400 degrees F" and timer to 23 minutes

5. Let it pre-heat until you hear a beep

6. Arrange chicken directly inside your cooking pot and lock lid, cook for 15 minutes, flip and cook for the remaining time

7. Serve and enjoy with yogurt dip!

Nutrition:

Calories: 321, Fat: 24 g, Saturated Fat: 5 g, Carbohydrates: 6 g, Fiber: 2 g, Sodium: 602 mg, Protein: 21 g

Chicken Zucchini Kebabs

Prep Time: 5-10 minutes

Cooking Time: 15 minutes

Serves: 4

Ingredients:

- Juice of 4 lemons
- Grated zest of 1 lemon
- 1-pound boneless, skinless chicken breasts, cut into cubes of 2 inches
- 1 teaspoon sea salt
- ½ teaspoon ground black pepper
- 2 tablespoons plain Greek yogurt
- ¼ cup extra-virgin olive oil
- 1 red onion, quartered
- 1 zucchini, sliced
- 4 garlic cloves, minced
- 2 tablespoons dried oregano

Directions:

1. In a mixing bowl, add the Greek yogurt, oil, lemon juice, zest, garlic, oregano, salt, and pepper. Combine the ingredients to mix well with each other.

2. Add the chicken and coat well. Refrigerate for 1-2 hours to marinate.

3. Take Ninja Foodi Grill, arrange it over your kitchen platform, and open the top lid.

4. Arrange the grill grate and close the top lid.

5. Press "GRILL" and select the "MED" grill function. Adjust the timer to 14 minutes and then press "START/STOP." Ninja Foodi will start pre-heating.

6. Take the skewers, thread the chicken, red onion, and zucchini. Thread alternatively.

7. Ninja Foodi is preheated and ready to cook when it starts to beep. After you hear a beep, open the top lid.

8. Arrange the skewers over the grill grate.

9. Close the top lid and allow it to cook until the timer reads zero. Baste the kebabs with a marinating mixture in between. Cook until the food thermometer reaches 165°F.

10. Serve warm.

Nutrition:

Calories: 277, Fat: 15.5g, Saturated Fat: 2g, Trans Fat: 0g, Carbohydrates: 9.5g, Fiber: 2g, Sodium: 523mg, Protein: 25g

Delicious Maple Glazed Chicken

Prep Time: 10 minutes

Cooking Time: 15 minutes

Serves: 4

Ingredients:

- 2 pounds chicken wings, bone-in
- 1 teaspoon black pepper, ground
- ¼ cup teriyaki sauce
- 1 cup maple syrup
- 1/3 cup soy sauce

- 3 garlic cloves, minced
- 2 teaspoons garlic powder
- 2 teaspoons onion powder

Directions:

1. Take a mixing bowl, add garlic, soy sauce, black pepper, maple syrup, garlic powder, onion powder, and teriyaki sauce, combine well
2. Add the chicken wings and combine well to coat
3. Arrange the grill grate and close the lid
4. Pre-heat Ninja Foodi by pressing the "GRILL" option and setting it to "MED" and timer to 10 minutes
5. Let it pre-heat until you hear a beep
6. Arrange the chicken wings over the grill grate lock lid and cook for 5 minutes
7. Flip the chicken and close the lid, cook for 5 minutes more
8. Cook until it reaches 165 degrees F
9. Serve warm and enjoy!

Nutrition:

Calories: 543, Fat: 26 g, Saturated Fat: 6 g, Carbohydrates: 46 g, Fiber: 4 g, Sodium: 648 mg, Protein: 42 g

Fried Chicken Thighs

Prep Time: 10 Minutes

Cooking Time: 25 Minutes

Servings: 4

Ingredients:

- 1/2 cup all-purpose flour
- egg, beaten
- 4 small chicken thighs
- 1 1/2 tablespoon Old Bay Cajun Seasoning
- 1 teaspoon seasoning salt

Directions:

1. Preheat the air fryer to 390 degrees F.
2. Mix flour with Old Bay and salt in a bowl.
3. Coat chicken with the dry mixture and shake off the excess.
4. Place the chicken thighs in the air fryer basket.
5. Cook for 25 minutes until golden brown.
6. Serve warm.

Nutrition:

Calories 180, Total Fat 20 g, Saturated Fat 5 g, Cholesterol 151 mg, Sodium 686 mg, Total Carbs 13 g, Fiber 1 g, Sugar 1.2 g, Protein 21 g

Chicken Chili and Beans

Prep Time: 10 minutes

Cooking Time: 15 minutes

Serves: 4

Ingredients:

- 1 and ¼ pounds chicken breast, cut into pieces
- 1 can black beans, drained and rinsed
- 1 tablespoon oil
- 1 can corn
- 1 bell pepper, chopped
- ¼ teaspoon garlic powder
- ¼ teaspoon garlic powder
- 2 tablespoons chili powder
- ¼ teaspoon salt

Directions:

1. Pre-heat Ninja Foodi by squeezing the "AIR CRISP" alternative and setting it to "360 Degrees F" and timer to 15 minutes
2. Place all the ingredients in your Ninja Foodi Grill cooking basket/alternatively, you may use a dish to mix the ingredients and then put the dish in the cooking basket

3. Stir to mix well

4. Cook for 15 minutes

5. Serve and enjoy!

Nutrition:

Calories: 220, Fat: 4 g, Saturated Fat: 1 g, Carbohydrates: 24 g, Fiber: 2 g, Sodium: 856 mg, Protein: 20 g

Sweet and Sour Chicken BBQ

Prep Time: 10 minutes

Cooking Time: 40 minutes

Serves: 4

Ingredients:

- 6 chicken drumsticks
- 1 cup of soy sauce
- 1 cup of water
- 1 cup white vinegar
- ¾ cup of sugar
- ¾ cup onion, minced
- ¼ cup tomato paste
- ¼ cup garlic, minced
- Salt and pepper, to taste

Directions:

1. Take a Ziploc bag and add all ingredients into it

2. Marinate for at least 2 hours in your refrigerator

3. Insert the crisper basket, and close the hood

4. Pre-heat Ninja Foodi by squeezing the "AIR CRISP" alternative at 390 degrees F for 40 minutes

5. Place the grill pan accessory in the Ninja Foodi Grill

6. Flip the chicken after every 10 minutes

7. Take a saucepan and pour the marinade into it and heat over medium flame until sauce thickens

8. Brush with the glaze

9. Serve warm and enjoy!

Nutrition:

Calories: 460, Fat: 20 g, Saturated Fat: 5 g, Carbohydrates: 26 g, Fiber: 3 g, Sodium: 126 mg, Protein: 28 g

Turkey Tomato Burgers

Prep Time: 5-10 minutes

Cooking Time: 40 minutes

Serves: 6

Ingredients:

- 2/3 cup sun-dried tomatoes, chopped
- 1/4 teaspoon salt
- 1 cup crumbled feta cheese
- 2 pounds lean ground turkey
- 1/4 teaspoon pepper
- 1 large red onion, chopped
- 6 burger buns of your choice, sliced in half

Directions:

1. In a mixing bowl, add all the ingredients. Combine the ingredients to mix well with each other.

2. Prepare six patties from the mixture.

3. Take Ninja Foodi Grill, arrange it over your kitchen platform, and open the top lid.

4. Arrange the grill grate and close the top lid.

5. Press "GRILL" and select the "MED" grill function. Adjust the timer to 14 minutes and then press "START/STOP." Ninja Foodi will start pre-heating.

6. Ninja Foodi is preheated and ready to cook when it starts to beep. After you hear a beep, open the top lid.

7. Arrange the patties over the grill grate.

8. Close the top lid and cook for 7 minutes. Now open the top lid, flip the patties.

9. Close the top lid and cook for 7 more minutes.

10. Serve warm with ciabatta rolls. Add your choice of toppings: lettuce, tomato, cheese, ketchup, cheese, etc.

Nutrition:

Calories: 298, Fat: 16g, Saturated Fat: 2.5g, Trans Fat: 0g, Carbohydrates: 32g, Fiber: 4g, Sodium: 321mg, Protein: 27.5g

Lemon Roasted Chicken

Prep Time: 10 minutes

Cooking Time: 55 minutes

Servings: 4

Ingredients:

- 2 tbsp. olive oil
- 2 tbsp. butter softened
- lemon, zested and juiced
- 4 garlic cloves, minced
- Salt and black pepper to taste
- 1 (3 lbs.) whole chicken

Directions:

7. Insert the dripping pan onto the bottom of the air fryer and preheat the device at Roast mode at 400 F for 2 to 3 minutes.

8. In a small bowl, mix the olive oil, butter, lemon zest, lemon juice, garlic, salt, and black pepper. Pat, the chicken, dries with paper towels, and rub the seasoning mix all around and inside the cavity of the chicken. Use cooking twines to tie and secure the wings, legs, and any loose ends into the body of the chicken.

9. Run the rotisserie spit through one open end of the chicken through to the other end and lock the forks with their screws.

10. Lift the chicken, lock the spit onto the lever in the Grill, and close the lid.

11. Set the timer to 50 minutes and press Start. Cook until the chicken is golden brown all around, and the meat is tender and almost falling off the bone.

12. When done cooking, open the Grill and use the rotisserie lift to remove the chicken off the lever.

13. Unscrew, pull out the spit, and allow the chicken to sit for 3 to 5 minutes before slicing and serving.

Nutrition:

Calories 296, Total Fat 16.81g, Total Carbs 2.89g, Fiber 0.3g, Protein 32.39g

Baked Coconut Chicken

Prep Time: 10 minutes

Cooking Time: 12 minutes

Serves: 4

Ingredients:

- 2 large eggs
- 2 teaspoons garlic powder
- 1 teaspoon salt
- ½ teaspoon ground black pepper
- ¾ cup coconut aminos
- 1-pound chicken tenders
- Cooking spray as needed

Directions:

1. Pre-heat Ninja Foodi by squeezing the "AIR CRISP" alternative and setting it to "400 Degrees F" and timer to 12 minutes

2. Take a large-sized baking sheet and spray it with cooking spray

3. Take a wide dish and add garlic powder, eggs, pepper, and salt

4. Whisk well until everything is combined

5. Add the almond meal and coconut and mix well

6. Take your chicken tenders and dip them in the egg followed by dipping in the coconut mix

7. Shake off any excess

8. Transfer them to your Ninja Foodi Grill and spray the tenders with a bit of oil.

9. Cook for 12-14 minutes until you have a nice golden-brown texture

10. Enjoy!

Nutrition:

Calories: 180, Fat: 1 g, Saturated Fat: 0 g, Carbohydrates: 3 g, Fiber: 1 g, Sodium: 214 mg, Protein: 0 g

Hot and Sassy BBQ Chicken

Prep Time: 5-10 minutes

Cooking Time: 18 minutes

Serves: 4

Ingredients:

- 2 tablespoons honey
- 2 cups BBQ sauce
- 1 tablespoon hot sauce
- 1-pound chicken drumstick
- Juice of 1 lime
- Pepper and salt as needed

Directions:

1. Take a bowl and add BBQ sauce, lime juice, honey, pepper, salt, hot sauce, and mix well

2. Take another mixing bowl and add ½ cup sauce and chicken mix well and add remaining ingredients

3. Let it sit for 1 hour to marinate

4. Pre-heat Ninja Foodi by pressing the "GRILL" option and setting it to "MED" and timer to 18 minutes

5. Let it pre-heat until you hear a beep

6. Arrange chicken over grill grate, cook until the timer reaches zero and internal temperature reaches 165 degrees F

7. Serve and enjoy!

Nutrition:

Calories: 423, Fat: 13 g, Saturated Fat: 6 g, Carbohydrates: 47 g, Fiber: 4 g, Sodium: 698 mg, Protein: 22 g

Grilled Orange Chicken

Prep Time: 5-10 minutes

Cooking Time: 10 minutes

Serves: 5-6

Ingredients:

- 1/2 teaspoon garlic salt
- 2 teaspoons ground coriander
- 12 chicken wings
- 1/4 teaspoon ground black pepper
- 1 tablespoon canola oil

Sauce:

- 1/4 cup butter, melted
- 3 tablespoons honey
- 1/2 cup orange juice
- 1/3 cup Sriracha chili sauce
- 2 tablespoons lime juice
- 1/4 cup chopped cilantro

Directions:

1. Coat chicken with oil and season with the spices; refrigerate for 2 hours to marinate.
2. Combine all the sauce ingredients and set aside. Optionally, you can stir-cook the sauce mixture for 3-4 minutes in a saucepan.
3. Take Ninja Foodi Grill, organize it over your kitchen stage, and open the top cover.
4. Organize the barbecue mesh and close the top cover.

5. Click "GRILL" and choose the "MED" grill function. Adjust the timer to 10 minutes and afterward press "START/STOP." Ninja Foodi will begin pre-warming.

6. Ninja Foodi is preheated and prepared to cook when it begins to signal. After you hear a blare, open the top.

7. Organize chicken over the grill grate.

8. Close the top lid and cook for 5 minutes. Now open the top lid, flip the chicken.

9. Close the top lid and cook for 5 more minutes.

Nutrition:

Calories: 327, Fat: 14g, Saturated Fat: 3.5g, Trans Fat: 0g, Carbohydrates: 19g, Fiber: 1g, Sodium: 258mg, Protein: 25g

Chapter 4: Appetizers & Snacks

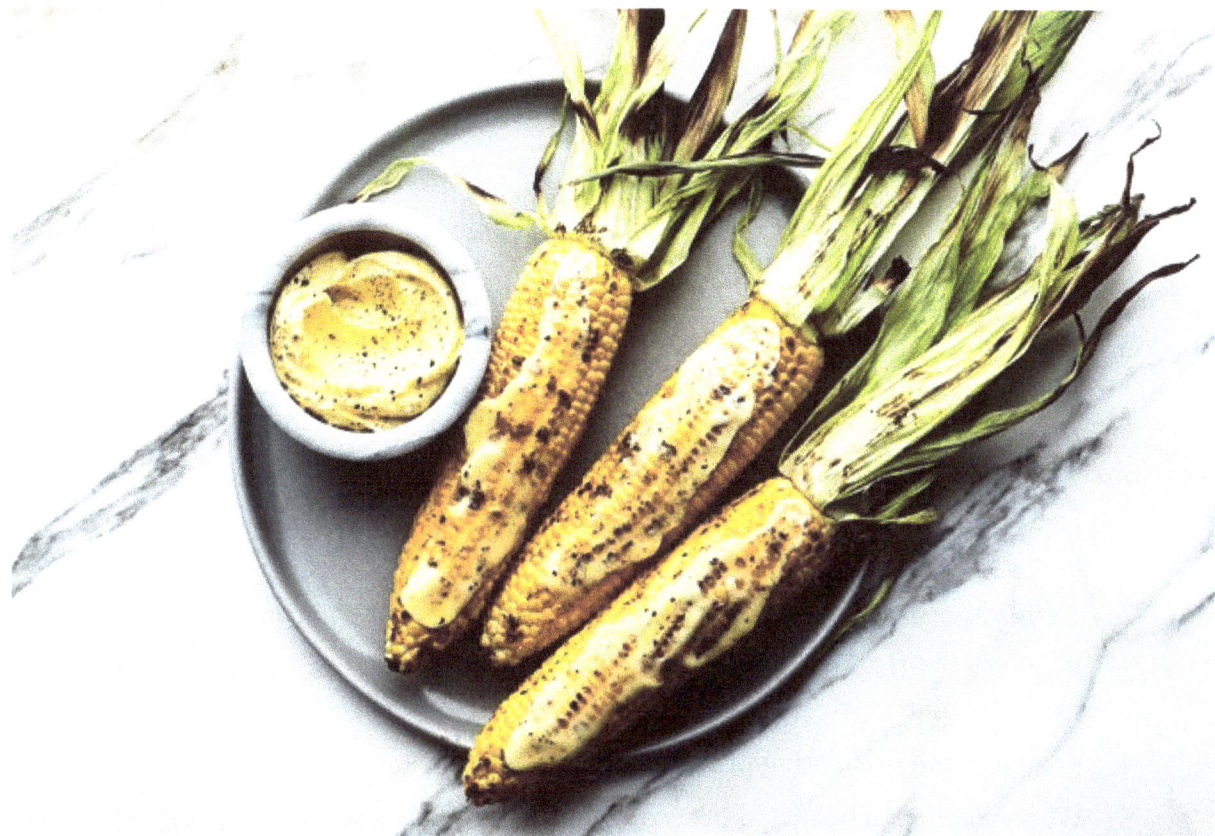

Delicious Grilled Honey Fruit Salad

- Prep time: 5-10 minutes

Cooking time: 5 minutes

Servings: 4

Ingredients:

- 1 tablespoon lime juice, freshly squeezed
- 6 tablespoons honey, divided
- 2 peaches, pitted and sliced
- 1 can (9 ounces) pineapple chunks, drained and juiced reserved
- ½ pound strawberries washed, hulled, and halved

Directions:

1. Take a shallow mixing bowl, then add respectively soy sauce, balsamic vinegar, oil, maple syrup and whisk well
2. Then add broccoli and keep it aside
3. Press the "GRILL" of the Ninja Foodi Grill and set it to "MAX" mode with 10 minutes timer
4. Keep it in the preheating process
5. When you hear a beat, add broccoli over the grill grate
6. After then lock the lid and cook until the timer shows 0
7. Lastly, garnish the food with pepper flakes and sesame seeds
8. Enjoy!

Nutrition:

Calories: 141, Fat: 7 g, Carbohydrate: 14 g, Protein: 4 g, Sodium: 853 mg, Fiber: 4 g, Saturated Fat: 1 g

7.

Ninja Grill Hot Dogs

Prep Time: 10 minutes

Cooking Time: 12 minutes

Serves: 4

Ingredients:

- 1 cup cabbage slaw

- 4 bacon slices, crispy
- 4 hot dogs
- 1/8 cup onion, chopped
- 4 hot dog buns, cut in half

Directions:

1. Sear the bacon in a skillet until crispy from both the sides.
2. Wrap a bacon strip around each hot dog and secure it by inserting a toothpick.
3. Prepare and preheat the Ninja Foodi Grill in a High-temperature setting.
4. Once it is preheated, open the lid and place 2 hot dogs in the grill.
5. Cover the Ninja Foodi Grill's lid and grill on the "Grilling Mode" for 6 minutes while rotating after every 2 minutes.
6. Cook all the hot dogs in batches then remove the toothpick.
7. Serve warm in a hotdog bun with cabbage slaw and onion.
8. Enjoy.

Nutrition:

Calories 301, Total Fat 32.2 g, Saturated Fat 2.4 g, Cholesterol 110 mg, Sodium 276 mg, Total Carbs 25 g, Fiber 0.9 g, Sugar 31.4 g, Protein 28.8 g

Broccoli Maple Grill

- Prep time: 5-10 minutes

Cooking time: 10 minutes
Servings:c4
Ingredients:

- 2 teaspoons maple syrup
- 4 tablespoon balsamic vinegar
- 2 tablespoon canola oil
- 4 tablespoons soy sauce
- 2 heads broccoli, cut into floret
- Pepper flakes and sesame seeds for garnish

Directions:

1. Take a shallow mixing bowl, then add respectively soy sauce, balsamic vinegar, oil, maple syrup and whisk well

2. Then add broccoli and keep it aside

3. Press the "GRILL" of the Ninja Foodi Grill and set it to "MAX" mode with 10 minutes timer

4. Keep it in the preheating process

5. When you hear a beat, add broccoli over the grill grate

6. After then lock the lid and cook until the timer shows 0

7. Lastly, garnish the food with pepper flakes and sesame seeds

8. Enjoy!

Nutrition:
Calories: 141, Fat: 7 g, Carbohydrate: 14 g, Protein: 4 g, Sodium: 853 mg, Fiber: 4 g, Saturated Fat: 1 g

8.

Grilled Eggplant

Prep Time: 10 minutes

Cooking Time: 10 minutes

Serves: 4

Ingredients:

- 2 small eggplants, half-inch slices
- 3 teaspoons Cajun seasoning
- 2 tablespoons lime juice
- 1/4 cup olive oil

Directions:

1. Liberally season the eggplant slices with oil, lemon juice, and Cajun seasoning.

2. Prepare and preheat the Ninja Foodi Grill on the medium temperature setting.

3. Once it is preheated, open the lid and place the eggplant slices in the grill.

4. Cover the Ninja Foodi Grill's lid and grill on the "Grilling Mode" for 5 minutes per side.

5. Serve.

Nutrition:

Calories 372, Total Fat 11.1 g, Saturated Fat 5.8 g, Cholesterol 610 mg, Sodium 749 mg, Total Carbs 16.9 g, Fiber 0.2 g, Sugar 0.2 g, Protein 13.5 g

Pineapple with Cream Cheese Dip

Prep Time: 10 minutes

Cooking Time: 8 minutes

Serves: 4

Ingredients:

DIP:

- 2 tablespoons honey
- 1 tablespoon brown sugar
- 3 oz. cream cheese, softened
- 1 tablespoon lime juice
- 1/4 cup yogurt
- 1 teaspoon grated lime zest

Pineapple:

- 1 fresh pineapple
- 3 tablespoons honey
- 2 tablespoons lime juice
- 1/4 cup packed brown sugar

Directions:

1. First, slice the peeled pineapple into 8 wedges then cut each wedge into 2 spears.
2. Toss the pineapple with sugar, lime juice, and honey in a bowl then refrigerate for 1 hour.
3. Meanwhile, prepare the lime dip by whisking all its ingredients together in a bowl.
4. Remove the pineapple from its marinade.
5. Prepare and preheat the Ninja Foodi Grill on the medium temperature setting.
6. Once it is preheated, open the lid and place the pineapple on the grill.

7. Cover the Ninja Foodi Grill's lid and grill on the "Grilling Mode" for 4 minutes per side.

8. Serve with lime dip.

Nutrition:

Calories 368, Total Fat 6 g, Saturated Fat 1.2 g, Cholesterol 351 mg, Sodium 103 mg, Total Carbs 72.8 g, Fiber 9.2 g, Sugar 32.9 g, Protein 7.2 g

Chicken Salad with Blueberry Vinaigrette

Prep Time: 10 minutes

Cooking Time: 14 minutes

Serves: 4

Ingredients:

- 2 boneless skinless chicken breasts, halves
- 1 tablespoon olive oil
- 1 garlic clove, minced
- 1/4 teaspoon salt
- 1/4 teaspoon pepper

Vinaigrette:

- 1/4 cup olive oil
- 1/4 cup blueberry preserves
- 2 tablespoons balsamic vinegar
- 2 tablespoons maple syrup
- 1/4 teaspoon ground mustard
- 1/8 teaspoon salt
- Dash pepper

Salads:

- 1 package (10 oz. salad greens
- 1 cup fresh blueberries
- 1/2 cup canned oranges

- 1 cup crumbled goat cheese

Directions:

1. First season the chicken liberally with garlic, salt, pepper and oil in a bowl.
2. Cover to refrigerate for 30 minutes margination.
3. Prepare and preheat the Ninja Foodi Grill on the medium temperature setting.
4. Once it is preheated, open the lid and place the chicken in the grill.
5. Cover the Ninja Foodi Grill's lid and grill on the "Grilling Mode" for 5-7 minutes per side until the internal temperature reaches 330 degrees F.
6. Toss the remaining ingredients for salad and vinaigrette in a bowl.
7. Slice the grilled chicken and serve with salad.

Nutrition:

Calories 379, Total Fat 29.7 g, Saturated Fat 18.6 g, Cholesterol 141 mg, Sodium 193 mg, Total Carbs 23.7g, Fiber 0.9 g, Sugar 19.3 g, Protein 5.2 g

Honey Glazed Bratwurst

Prep Time: 10 minutes

Cooking Time: 10 minutes

Serves: 4

Ingredients:

- 4 bratwurst links, uncooked
- 1/4 cup Dijon mustard
- 4 brat buns, split
- 2 tablespoons mayonnaise
- 1 teaspoon steak sauce
- 1/4 cup honey

Directions:

1. First, mix the mustard with steak sauce and mayonnaise in a bowl.
2. Prepare and preheat the Ninja Foodi Grill on a High-temperature setting.
3. Once it is preheated, open the lid and place the bratwurst on the grill.

4. Cover the Ninja Foodi Grill's lid and grill on the "Grilling Mode" for 10 minutes per side until their internal temperature reaches 320 degrees F.

5. Serve with buns and mustard sauce on top.

Nutrition:

Calories 213, Total Fat 14 g, Saturated Fat 8 g, Cholesterol 81 mg, Sodium 162 mg, Total Carbs 53 g, Fiber 0.7 g, Sugar 19 g, Protein 12 g

Creamed Potato Corns

- Prep time: 5-10 minutes

Cooking time: 30-40 minutes

Servings: 4

Ingredients:

- 1 and ½ teaspoon garlic salt
- ½ cup sour cream
- 1 jalapeno pepper, seeded and minced
- 1 tablespoon lime juice
- 1 teaspoon ground cumin
- ½ cup milk
- 2 poblano pepper
- ¼ teaspoon cayenne pepper
- 2 sweet corn years
- 1 tablespoon cilantro, minced
- 3 tablespoons olive oil

Directions:

1. Drain potatoes and rub them with oil
2. Pre-heat your Ninja Foodi Grill to MED, setting a timer for 10 minutes
3. Once you hear the beep, arrange poblano peppers over the grill grate
4. Let them cook for 5 minutes, flip and cook for 5 minutes more
5. Grill remaining veggies in the same way, giving 7 minutes to each side
6. Take a bowl and whisk in the remaining ingredients and prepare your vinaigrette
7. Peel grilled corn and chop them

8. Divide ears into small pieces and cut the potatoes

9. Serve grilled veggies with vinaigrette

10. Enjoy!

Nutrition:

Calories: 344, Fat: 5 g, Saturated Fat: 1 g, Carbohydrates: 51 g, Fiber: 3 g, Sodium: 600 mg, Protein: 5 g

Fully Grilled Sweet Honey Carrot

- Prep time: 10 minutes

Cooking time: 10 minutes

Servings: 6

Ingredients:

- 1 teaspoon salt

- 1 tablespoon honey

- 1 tablespoon rosemary, chopped

- 1 tablespoon parsley, chopped

- 6 carrots, cut lengthwise

- 2 tablespoons butter, melted

Directions:

1. Pre-heat your Ninja Foodi Grill to MAX, set a timer for 10 minutes

2. Once you hear the beep, arrange carrots over the grill grate

3. Spread remaining ingredients and drizzle honey

4. Lock lid and cook for 5 minutes, flip and cook for 5 minutes more

5. Serve and enjoy!

Tarragon Asparagus

Prep Time: 10 minutes

Cooking Time: 16 minutes

Serves: 4

Ingredients:

- 2 lbs. fresh asparagus, trimmed

- 1/2 teaspoon pepper
- 1/4 cup honey
- 2 tablespoons olive oil
- 1 teaspoon salt
- 4 tablespoons minced fresh tarragon

Directions:

1. Liberally season the asparagus by tossing with oil, salt, pepper, honey, and tarragon.
2. Prepare and preheat the Ninja Foodi Grill on the medium temperature setting.
3. Once it is preheated, open the lid and place the asparagus on the grill.
4. Cover the Ninja Foodi Grill's lid and grill on the "Grilling Mode" for 8 minutes per side, give them a toss after 4 minutes.
5. Serve warm.

Nutrition:

Calories 248, Total Fat 15.7 g, Saturated Fat 2.7 g, Cholesterol 75 mg, Sodium 94 mg, Total Carbs 31.4 g, Fiber 0.6 g, Sugar 15 g, Protein 14.1 g

Grilled Butternut Squash

Prep Time: 10 minutes

Cooking Time: 16 minutes

Serves: 4

Ingredients:

- 1 teaspoon dried thyme
- 1 medium butternut squash
- 1 tablespoon olive oil
- 1/2 teaspoon salt
- 1 ½ teaspoons dried oregano
- 1/4 teaspoon pepper

Directions:

1. Peel and slice the squash into ½ inch thick slices.

2. Remove the center of the slices to discard the seeds.

3. Toss the squash slices with remaining ingredients in a bowl.

4. Prepare and preheat the Ninja Foodi Grill on the medium temperature setting.

5. Once it is preheated, open the lid and place the squash in the grill.

6. Cover the Ninja Foodi Grill's lid and grill on the "Grilling Mode" for 8 minutes per side.

7. Serve warm.

Nutrition:

Calories 249, Total Fat 11.9 g, Saturated Fat 1.7 g, Cholesterol 78 mg, Sodium 79 mg, Total Carbs 41.8 g, Fiber 1.1 g, Sugar 20.3 g, Protein 15 g

9.

Complete Italian Squash

- Prep time: 5-10 minutes

Cooking time: 16 minutes
Servings: 4
Ingredients:

- ¼ teaspoon black pepper

- 1 and ½ teaspoons dried oregano

- 1 tablespoon olive oil

- ½ teaspoon salt

- 1 teaspoon dried thyme

- 1 medium butternut squash, peeled, seeded, and cut into ½ inch slices

Directions:

1. Take a mixing bowl and add slices and other ingredients, mix well

2. Pre-heat your Ninja Foodi Grill to MED and set the timer to 16 minutes

3. Once you hear the beep, arrange squash slices over the grill grate

4. Cook for 8 minutes, flip and cook for 8 minutes

5. Serve and enjoy!

Nutrition:
Calories: 238, Fat: 12 g, Saturated Fat: 2 g, Carbohydrates: 36 g, Fiber: 3 g, Sodium: 128 mg, Protein: 15 g

10.

Lovely Seasonal Broccoli

- Prep time: 10 minutes

Cooking time: 10 minutes

Servings: 4

Ingredients:

- ½ teaspoon salt
- ½ teaspoon red chili powder
- ¼ teaspoon spice mix
- 2 tablespoons yogurt
- 1 tablespoon chickpea flour
- ¼ teaspoon turmeric powder
- 1 pound broccoli, cut into florets

Directions:

1. Take your florets and wash them thoroughly
2. Take a bowl and add listed ingredients, except the florets
3. Add broccoli and combine the mix well; let the mixture sit for 30 minutes
4. Pre-heat your Ninja Foodi to AIR CRISP mode at 390 degrees F and set the timer to 10 minutes
5. Once you hear a beep, add florets and crisp for 10 minutes
6. Serve and enjoy once done!

Nutrition:

Calories: 111, Fat: 2 g, Saturated Fat: 1 g, Carbohydrates: 12 g, Fiber: 1 g, Sodium: 024 mg, Protein: 7 g

Mammamia Banana Boats

- Prep time: 19 minutes

Cooking time: 6 minutes

Servings: 4

Ingredients:

- ½ cup peanut butter chips
- ½ cup of chocolate chips
- 1 cup mini marshmallows

- 4 ripe bananas

Directions:

1. With the peel, slice a banana lengthwise and remember that not to cut all the way through.

2. Onward, reveal the inside of the banana by using your hand

3. Press the "GRILL" option and set this in "MEDIUM" to pre-heat Ninja Foodi with a 6 minutes timer

4. Until you hear a beep, keep it in the pre-heat process

5. Put the banana over the Grill Grate and lock the lid, let it cook for 4-6 minutes until chocolate melts and bananas are toasted

6. Serve and Enjoy!

Nutrition:
Calories: 505, Fat: 18 g, Carbohydrates: 82 g, Protein: 10 g, Sodium: 166 mg, Fiber: 6 g, Saturated Fat: 4 g

Cob with Pepper Butter

Prep Time: 10 minutes

Cooking Time: 30 minutes

Serves: 8

Ingredients:

- 1 cup butter, softened

- 8 medium ears sweet corn

- 2 tablespoons lemon-pepper seasoning

Directions:

1. Season the corn cob with butter and lemon pepper liberally.

2. Prepare and preheat the Ninja Foodi Grill on a medium-temperature setting.

3. Once it is preheated, open the lid and place the corn cob in the grill.

4. Cover the Ninja Foodi Grill's lid and grill on the "Grilling Mode" for 15 minutes while rotating after every 5 minutes.

5. Grill the corn cobs in batches.

6. Serve warm.

Nutrition:

Calories 148, Total Fat 22.4 g, Saturated Fat 10.1 g, Cholesterol 320 mg, Sodium 350 mg, Total Carbs 32.2 g, Fiber 0.7 g, Sugar 0.7 g, Protein 4.3 g

Chapter 5: Meat

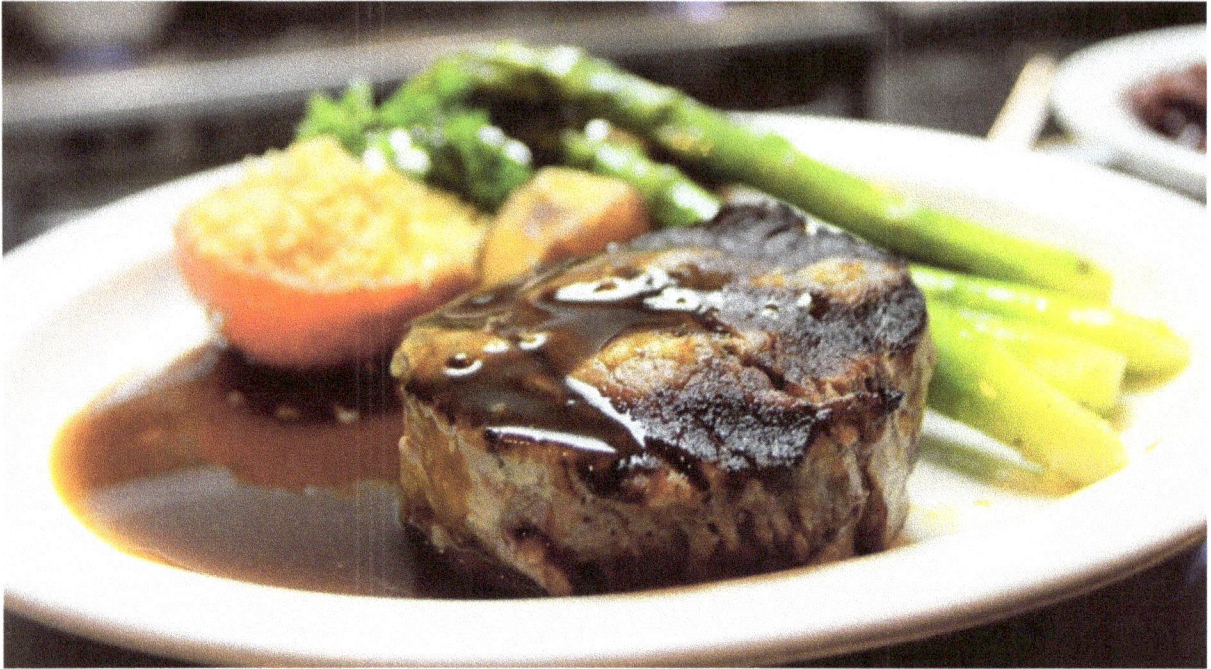

Sausage & Pepper

Prep Time: 30 minutes

Cooking Time: 20 minutes

Serves: 6

Ingredients:

- 1 white onion, sliced into rings
- 2 tablespoons vegetable oil
- 6 Italian sausages
- Salt and pepper to taste
- 2 bell peppers, sliced

Directions:

1. Add grill grate to your Ninja Foodi Grill.
2. Close the hood.
3. Choose grill setting.

4. Set it to low. Set it to 25 minutes. Press start to preheat.

5. Toss onions and bell peppers in oil.

6. Season with salt and pepper.

7. Add veggies to the grill grate.

8. Cook for 10 minutes.

9. Transfer veggies to a bowl.

10. Grill sausages for 5 minutes per side.

11. Top sausages with veggies.

Serving Suggestions: Serve as is or in hot dog buns.

Preparation / Cooking Tips: You can also use Bratwurst for this recipe.

Roast Beef with Garlic

Prep Time: 15 minutes

Cooking Time: 1 hour and 20 minutes

Serves: 4

Ingredients:

- 2 lb. beef roast, sliced
- 6 cloves garlic
- Salt and pepper to taste
- 2 tablespoons vegetable oil

Directions:

1. Coat beef roast with oil.

2. Season with salt and pepper.

3. Place inside the Ninja Foodi Grill pot.

4. Sprinkle garlic on top.

5. Choose bake setting.

6. Set it to 400 degrees F and cook for 30 minutes.

7. Reduce temperature to 375 degrees F and cook for another 40 minutes.

Serving Suggestions: Serve with mashed potato and gravy.

Preparation / Cooking Tips: If refrigerated, let beef come to room temperature 2 hours before cooking.

Ranch Pork Chops

Prep Time: 20 minutes

Cooking Time: 20 minutes

Serves: 4

Ingredients:

- 1 teaspoon garlic powder
- 1 tablespoon Parmesan cheese, grated
- 1/2 cup ranch dressing
- Salt and pepper to taste
- 1 cup breadcrumbs
- 1 tablespoon buttermilk
- 4 pork chops

Directions:

1. Mix garlic powder, breadcrumbs, Parmesan cheese, salt and pepper in a bowl.
2. Combine buttermilk and ranch dressing in another wall.
3. Dip the pork chops in the buttermilk mixture.
4. Dredge with the breadcrumb mixture.
5. Set the Ninja Foodi Grill to air crisp.
6. Cook at 330 degrees F for 10 minutes per side.

Serving Suggestions: Serve with vegetable salad.

Preparation / Cooking Tips: You can also use other types of milk for this recipe.

Steak Kebab

Prep Time: 30 minutes

Cooking Time: 15 minutes

Serves: 4

Ingredients:

- 8 button mushrooms
- 1 white onion, sliced into wedges
- 2 strip steaks, sliced into cubes
- 1 bell pepper, sliced
- Dash steak seasoning
- Salt and pepper to taste

Directions:

1. Add grill grate to the Ninja Foodi Grill.
2. Close the hood and press grill setting.
3. Set it to high. Set it to 12 minutes. Press start to preheat.
4. While waiting, thread steak and veggies onto skewers.
5. Season with steak seasoning, salt and pepper.
6. Place on top of the grill grate.
7. Cook for 8 minutes.
8. Flip and cook for another 6 to 7 minutes.

Serving Suggestions: Serve with brown rice.

Preparation / Cooking Tips: Brush with barbecue basting sauce halfway through grilling.

Cuban Pork Chops

Prep Time: 8 hours and 20 minutes

Cooking Time: 30 minutes

Serves: 4

Ingredients:

- 4 pork chops
- 1/2 cup olive oil
- 1/2 cup lime juice
- 1 teaspoon orange zest
- 8 cloves garlic, minced

- 1/4 cup mint leaves, chopped
- 2 teaspoons dried oregano
- 1 cup orange juice
- 1 teaspoon lime zest
- 2 teaspoons ground cumin
- 1 cup cilantro, chopped

Directions:

1. Place pork chops in a shallow plate.
2. In another bowl, mix the remaining ingredients.
3. Take ¼ cup of the mixture and set aside.
4. Add the remaining mixture to the pork chops.
5. Cover and marinate in the refrigerator for 8 hours.
6. Add grill grate to the Ninja Foodi Grill. Seal the hood.
7. Choose grill setting.
8. Set it to high.
9. Set the time to 15 minutes.
10. Close the hood and cook for 15 minutes, flipping once.

Serving Suggestions: Let rest for 5 minutes before slicing and serving.

Preparation / Cooking Tips: You can also marinate only for 1 hour if you want shorter preparation time.

Grilled Steak & Potatoes

Prep Time: 20 minutes

Cooking Time: 50 minutes

Serves: 4

Ingredients:

- 1/4 cup avocado oil
- 4 potatoes
- 2 tablespoons steak seasoning

- 3 sirloin steaks
- Salt to taste

Directions:

1. Poke potatoes with fork.
2. Coat potatoes with half of avocado oil.
3. Season with salt.
4. Add to the air fryer basket.
5. Choose air crisp function in your Ninja Foodi Grill.
6. Seal the hood and cook at 400 degrees F for 35 minutes.
7. Flip and cook for another 10 minutes.
8. Transfer to a plate.
9. Add grill grate to the Ninja Foodi Grill.
10. Add steaks to the grill grate.
11. Set it to high.
12. Cook for 7 minutes per side.
13. Serve steaks with potatoes.

Serving Suggestions: Serve with steak sauce and hot sauce.

Preparation / Cooking Tips: Press steaks onto the grill to give it grill marks.

Rib Eye Steak with Onions & Peppers

Prep Time: 20 minutes

Cooking Time: 20 minutes

Serves: 2

Ingredients:

- 1/2 teaspoon cumin
- 2 rib eye steaks
- 1 tablespoon vegetable oil
- 1 teaspoon smoked paprika
- 1/2 teaspoon onion powder

- 1 red bell pepper, sliced
- 1/2 teaspoon garlic powder
- Salt and pepper to taste
- 1 white onion, sliced into rings
- 1/4 cup fajita sauce

Directions:

1. Combine cumin, onion powder, garlic powder, paprika, salt and pepper to taste.
2. Add grill grate to your Ninja Foodi Grill.
3. Place the veggie tray on the grill grate. Seal the hood.
4. Choose grill setting.
5. Preheat it to medium for 20 minutes.
6. Coat steaks with half of oil.
7. Sprinkle with half of spice blend.
8. Toss the onions and bell pepper with remaining oil and spice blend.
9. Add steaks on the grill grate.
10. Cook for 10 minutes.
11. Brush both sides with fajita sauce.
12. Cook for another 10 minutes.
13. Add veggies to the veggie tray.
14. Cook with the steak for 10 minutes.

Serving Suggestions: Serve with fresh green salad or pasta.

Preparation / Cooking Tips: Increase cooking time if you want your steaks well-done.

Tenderloin Steak with Bacon

Prep Time: 15 minutes

Cooking Time: 20 minutes

Serves: 4

Ingredients:

- 8 bacon strips

- 2 tablespoons vegetable oil
- Salt and pepper to taste
- 4 tenderloin steaks

Directions:

1. Wrap the tenderloin steak with bacon strips.
2. Coat the steaks with oil.
3. Sprinkle with salt and pepper.
4. Insert grill grate in the Ninja Foodi Grill.
5. Choose grill setting.
6. Set it to high for 12 minutes.
7. Press start to preheat.
8. Add the steaks on the grill.
9. Cook for 6 to 8 minutes per side.

Serving Suggestions: Serve with side vegetable salad.

Preparation / Cooking Tips: You can use a toothpick to secure the bacon around the steaks.

Grilled Pork Chops

Prep Time: 10 minutes

Cooking Time: 15 minutes

Serves: 4

Ingredients:

- 4 pork chops
- Barbecue sauce
- Salt and pepper to taste

Directions:

1. Add grill grate to your Ninja Foodi Grill.
2. Set it to grill. Close the hood.
3. Preheat to high for 15 minutes.
4. Season pork chops with salt and pepper.

5. Add to the grill grates.

6. Grill for 8 minutes.

7. Flip and cook for another 7 minutes, brushing both sides with barbecue sauce.

Serving Suggestions: Let rest for 5 minutes before slicing and serving.

Preparation / Cooking Tips: You can also make your own barbecue sauce by mixing soy sauce, sugar or honey, lemon juice and ketchup.

Paprika Pork Chops

Prep Time: 15 minutes

Cooking Time: 15 minutes

Serves: 2

Ingredients:

- 2 pork chops
- Salt and pepper to taste
- 1 teaspoon smoked paprika
- 1 teaspoon garlic powder
- 1 teaspoon olive oil

Directions:

1. Brush pork chops with oil.

2. Sprinkle with paprika, garlic powder, salt and pepper.

3. Set your Ninja Foodi Grill to air crisp.

4. Add pork chops to the air fryer basket.

5. Cook at 360 degrees F for 15 minutes.

6. Flip and cook for another 15 minutes.

7. Let sit for 3 to 5 minutes before serving.

Serving Suggestions: Serve with cucumber and tomato slices.

Preparation / Cooking Tips: Marinate for 15 minutes before air frying.

Coffee Rib-eye

Prep Time: 20 minutes

Cooking Time: 30 minutes

Serves: 4

Ingredients:

- 1 teaspoon onion powder
- 4 rib eye steaks
- 1 tablespoon vegetable oil
- 2 tablespoons coffee
- 1 teaspoon garlic powder
- 2 tablespoons ground chipotle pepper
- 1/2 teaspoon ground ginger
- 1/2 teaspoon mustard powder
- Salt and pepper to taste

Directions:

1. Brush both sides of steak with oil.
2. In a bowl, mix the remaining ingredients.
3. Sprinkle steak with spice mixture.
4. Add grill grate to your Ninja Foodi Grill.
5. Seal the hood and choose grill setting.
6. Set it to high. Start to preheat.
7. Add grill to the grate.
8. Once the temperate reaches 11o degrees F, flip the beef.
9. Wait until the pot beeps.
10. Let it rest for 10 minutes before slicing and serving.

Serving Suggestions: Serve with steamed veggies.

Preparation / Cooking Tips: Press steaks to give it grill marks.

Roast Beef & Grilled Potatoes

Prep Time: 15 minutes

Cooking Time: 45 minutes

Serves: 6

Ingredients:

- 2 1/2 teaspoons onion powder
- 3 lb. top round roast
- 4 cups potatoes, grilled
- 2 1/2 teaspoons garlic powder
- Salt and pepper to taste

Directions:

1. Combine onion powder, garlic powder, salt and pepper in a bowl.
2. Rub top round roast with dry rub.
3. Set the Ninja Foodi Grill to broil.
4. Preheat it to high for 10 minutes.
5. Add the roast beef and cook for 25 minutes.
6. Turn and cook for another 20 minutes.
7. Serve with grilled potatoes.

Serving Suggestions: Slice against the grain and serve.

Preparation / Cooking Tips: Let the roast come to room temperature for 1 hour before seasoning.

Cheeseburger

Prep Time: 20 minutes

Cooking Time: 10 minutes

Serves: 4

Ingredients:

- 1 1/2 lb. ground beef
- 1 egg, beaten

- 1 tablespoon breadcrumbs
- 4 cheese slices
- 1 onion, minced
- Salt and pepper to taste
- 1 red bell pepper, chopped
- 4 burger buns

Directions:

1. Insert grill grate to your Ninja Foodi Grill.
2. Choose grill setting.
3. Set it to high. Set time to 10 minutes.
4. Preheat your unit.
5. In a bowl, mix ground beef, onion, bell pepper, breadcrumbs and egg.
6. Form patties from the mixture.
7. Season patties with salt and pepper.
8. Add patties to the grill.
9. Cook for 8 to 10 minutes.
10. Add cheese on top of the beef and cook for another 1 minute.
11. Serve patties and cheese on burger buns.

Serving Suggestions: Serve with desired condiments.

Preparation / Cooking Tips: Use lean ground beef.

Grilled Herbed Steak

Prep Time: 15 minutes

Cooking Time: 10 minutes

Serves: 4

Ingredients:

- 4 steaks
- 4 sprigs rosemary, chopped
- 1 teaspoon dried basil

- 1 teaspoon dried tarragon
- Garlic salt to taste

Directions:

1. Add grill grate to the Ninja Foodi Grill.
2. Close the hood and choose grill setting.
3. Set it to 15 minutes.
4. Set it to high.
5. Press start to preheat.
6. Rub both sides of steak with garlic salt.
7. Sprinkle with herbs.
8. Add steaks to the grill grate.
9. Cook for 5 minutes per side.

Serving Suggestions: Garnish with fresh rosemary sprig.

Preparation / Cooking Tips: Marinate steak in herbs for 15 minutes before cooking.

Steak with Asparagus

Prep Time: 20 minutes

Cooking Time: 20 minutes

Serves: 4

Ingredients:

- 2 strip steaks
- Pinch steak seasoning
- Salt and pepper to taste
- 2 tablespoons vegetable oil, divided
- 2 cups asparagus, trimmed and sliced

Directions:

1. Coat strip steaks with half of oil.
2. Season with steak seasoning, salt and pepper.
3. Toss asparagus with oil, salt and pepper.

4. Add grill grate to the Ninja Foodi Grill. Seal the hood.

5. Select grill function and preheat it to high for 10 minutes.

6. Add steaks to the grill.

7. Cook for 5 minutes.

8. Flip and cook for 5 more minutes.

9. Add asparagus to the veggie tray.

10. Place veggie tray on top of the grill grate.

11. Cook for 10 minutes.

12. Serve steak with asparagus.

Serving Suggestions: Serve with salad or brown rice.

Preparation / Cooking Tips: Press steaks onto the grill to give it grill marks.

Chapter 6: Vegetarian and Vegan

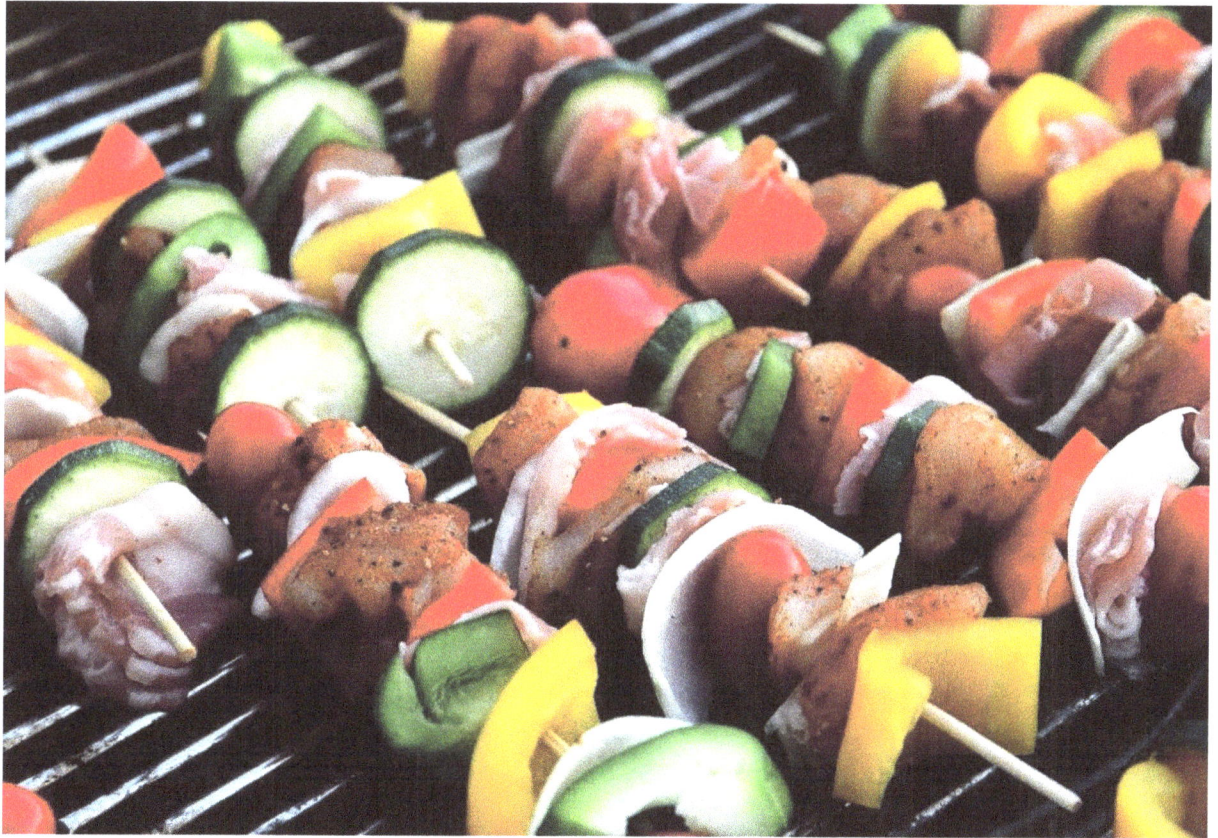

10.

Delicious Cajun Eggplant

Prep Time: 5-10 minutes

Cooking Time: 12 minutes

Servings: 4

Ingredients:

- ¼ cup olive oil
- 2 small eggplants, cut into slices
- 3 teaspoons Cajun seasoning
- 2 tablespoons lime juice

Directions:

8. Coat eggplant slices with oil, lemon juice, and Cajun seasoning

9. Take your Ninja Foodi Grill and press "GRILL" and set to "MED" mode, set the timer to 10 minutes

10. Let it preheat

11. Arrange eggplants over grill grate, lock lid and cook for 5 minutes

12. Flip and cook for 5 minutes more

13. Serve and enjoy!

Nutrition:

Calories: 362, Fat: 11 g, Saturated Fat: 3 g, Carbohydrates: 16 g, Fiber: 1 g, Sodium: 694 mg, Protein: 8 g

Cool Rosemary Potatoes

Prep Time: 10 minutes

Cooking Time: 20 minutes

Servings: 4

Ingredients:

- 2 pounds baby red potatoes, quartered
- ½ teaspoon parsley, dried
- ¼ teaspoon celery powder
- 2 tablespoons extra virgin olive oil
- ¼ cup onion flakes, dried
- ½ teaspoon garlic powder
- ½ teaspoon onion powder
- ½ teaspoon salt
- ¼ teaspoon freshly ground black pepper

Directions:

1. Add all listed ingredients into a large bowl

2. Toss well and coat them well

3. Pre-heat your Ninja Foodi by pressing the "AIR CRISP" option and setting it to 390 Degrees F

4. Set the timer to 20 minutes

5. Allow it to pre-heat until it beeps

6. Once preheated, add potatoes to the cooking basket

7. Close the lid and cook for 10 minutes

8. Shake the basket and cook for 10 minutes more

9. Check the crispness if it is done or not

10. Cook for 5 minutes more if needed

11. Serve and enjoy!

Nutrition:

Calories: 232, Fat: 7 g, Saturated Fat: 1 g, Carbohydrates: 39 g, Fiber: 6 g, Sodium: 249 mg, Protein: 4 g

Olive and Spinach Crispies

Prep time: 5 - 10 minutes

Cooking time: 15 minutes

Servings:

Ingredients:

- Salt and pepper to taste
- 4 teaspoons lemon zest, grated
- 2/3 cups Kalamata olives, halved and pitted
- 4 tablespoons butter
- 1 and ½ cups feta cheese, grated
- 2 pounds spinach, chopped and boiled

Directions:

1. Take a bowl and add butter, spinach, salt, and pepper; mix well

2. Pre-heat your Ninja Foodi Grill to 340 Degrees F in AIR CRISP mode, set the timer to 15 minutes

3. Once you hear the beep, arrange a reversible trivet in your Grill Pan

4. Arrange spinach mix in a basket in the trivet

5. Roast for 15 minutes, serve and enjoy!

Nutrition:

Calories: 250, Fat: 18 g, Saturated Fat: 3 g, Carbohydrates: 8 g, Fiber: 4 g, Sodium: 339 mg, Protein: 10 g

Definitive Air Brussels

Prep time: 5 - 10 minutes

Cooking time: 12 minutes

Servings: 4

Ingredients:

- ½ teaspoon pepper, ground
- 1 teaspoon salt
- 2 tablespoons olive oil, extra virgin
- 1-pound Brussels sprouts halved
- 6 slices bacon, chopped

Directions:

1. Take a bowl and add olive oil, Brussels, pepper and mix well
2. Pre-heat your Ninja Foodi to 390 degrees F in AIR CRISP mode, set the timer to 12 minutes
3. Once you hear the beep, arrange Brussels over the basket, cook for 6 minutes
4. Shake and cook for 6 minutes more
5. Serve and enjoy!

Nutrition:

Calories: 279, Fat: 18 g, Saturated Fat: 4 g, Carbohydrates: 12 g, Fiber: 4 g, Sodium: 874 mg

Mustard Dredged Veggie Delight

Prep Time: 5-10 minutes

Cooking Time: 30-40 minutes

Servings: 4

Ingredients:

Vinaigrette

- 2 tablespoons Dijon mustard
- ½ cup red wine vinegar
- 2 tablespoons honey
- 1 teaspoon salt
- ¼ teaspoon pepper
- ½ cup avocado oil
- ½ cup olive oil

Veggies

- 4 zucchinis, halved
- 4 sweet onion, quartered
- 4 red pepper, seeded and halved
- 2 bunch green onions, trimmed
- 4 yellow squash, cut in half

Directions:

1. Take a small-sized bowl and whisk in vinegar, mustard, honey, pepper, and salt. Add oils and combine well to make a smooth mixture
2. Preheat Ninja Foodi by pressing the "GRILL" option and setting it to "MED" and timer to 40 minutes
3. Let it preheat until you hear a beep
4. Arrange the onion quarters over the Grill Grate, lock lid, and cook for 5 minutes. Flip onions and cook for 5 minutes more
5. Grill remaining vegetables similarly, giving 7 minutes per side for the zucchini and pepper, and 1 minute per side for green onions
6. Serve the grilled vegetables with the mustard vinaigrette on top
7. Enjoy!

Nutrition:

Calories: 327, Fat: 5 g, Saturated Fat: 2 g, Carbohydrates:328 g, Fiber: 2 g, Sodium: 524 mg, Protein: 8 g

Zucchini and Egg Delight

Prep time: 10 minutes

Cooking time:8 minutes

Servings: 4

Ingredients:

- ½ teaspoon salt
- 1 teaspoon butter
- 1 zucchini, grated
- 2 tablespoons almond flour
- 4 whole eggs

Directions:

1. Take a mixing bowl and add almond flour, zucchini, salt. Mix well
2. Grease muffin molds with butter and adds zucchini mixture to them
3. Arrange muffin tins in your Ninja Foodi Grill and lock lid, lock lid and cook on "Air Crisp" mode for 7 minutes at 375 degrees F
4. Once done, take it out, serve, and enjoy!

Nutrition:

Calories: 94, Fat: 8 g, Saturated Fat: 1.5 g, Carbohydrates: 2 g, Fiber: 0.5 g, Sodium: 209 mg, Protein: 7 g

Premium Broccoli and Garlic Meal

Prep time: 5 - 10 minutes

Cooking time: 10 minutes

Servings: 4

Ingredients:

- 2 heads broccoli, cut into florets
- 4 tablespoon soy sauce
- 2 tablespoon canola oil
- 4 tablespoon balsamic vinegar

- 2 teaspoon maple syrup
- Red pepper flakes and sesame seeds for garnish

Directions:

6. First, take a mixing bowl and put vinegar, soy sauce, oil, maple syrup, and whisk, then mix all those ingredients.

7. Onward add broccoli to the mixture and keep them aside for a while.

8. Take your Ninja Foodi Grill and set this in the "MAX" mode with 10 minutes timer.

9. After hearing the first beep add the broccoli which was prepared before, over the Grill Grate.

10. Keep all those in the cooking process until the timer is 0.

11. Garnish with sesame seeds, pepper flakes if you like to taste spicy.

12. Enjoy.

Nutrition:

Calories: 141, Fat: 7g, Carbohydrate: 14g, Protein: 4g, Sodium: 853 mg, Fiber: 4g, Saturated Fat: 1g

Charred up Shishito Pepper

Prep Time: 10 minutes

Cooking Time: 10 minutes

Servings: 4

Ingredients:

- 3 cups Shishito peppers
- 2 tablespoons vegetable oil
- Salt and pepper to taste

Directions:

1. Select GRILL mode and set your Ninja Foodi Grill to "MAX," set timer to 10 minutes

2. Let it preheat until you hear a beep

3. Transfer pepper to grill grate and press peppers down, lock lid and cook for 8-10 minutes

4. Once done, serve with some salt and pepper sprinkled on top

5. Enjoy!

Nutrition:

Calories: 83, Fat: 7 g, Saturated Fat: 2 g, Carbohydrates: 5 g, Fiber: 1 g, Sodium: 49 mg, Protein: 2 g

The Creamy Potato Meal

Prep Time: 10 minutes

Cooking Time: 30- 40 minutes

Servings: 4

Ingredients:

- 1 and ½ pound red potatoes, quartered and boiled
- 3 tablespoons olive oil
- 1 tablespoon cilantro, minced
- 2 sweet corn ears, without husks
- ¼ teaspoon cayenne pepper
- 2 poblano pepper
- ½ cup milk
- 1 teaspoon ground cumin
- 1 tablespoon lime juice
- 1 jalapeno pepper, seeded and minced
- ½ cup sour cream
- 1 and ½ teaspoon garlic salt

Directions:

1. Drain the potatoes and rub them well with oil

2. Preheat Ninja Foodi by pressing the "GRILL" option and setting it to "MED" and timer to 10 minutes

3. Let it preheat until you hear a beep

4. Arrange your prepared poblano pepper over the grill grate, lock lid and cook for 5 minutes

5. Flip the peppers and cook for 5 minutes more

6. Grill the remaining vegetables in the same manner with 7 minutes each side for the potatoes and corn

7. Take a bowl and whisk in remaining ingredients to prepare the vinaigrette

8. Peel the grilled corn and chop

9. Divide corn ears into small pieces and cut your potatoes

10. Serve the grilled veggies with the vinaigrette topping

11. Enjoy!

Nutrition:

Calories: 344, Fat: 5 g, Saturated Fat: 1 g, Carbohydrates: 31 g, Fiber: 5 g, Sodium: 96 mg, Protein: 5 g

Corny Creamy Potatoes

Prep Time: 5-10 minutes

Cooking Time: 30-40 minutes

Servings: 4

Ingredients:

- 1 and ½ pound red potatoes, quartered and boiled
- 3 tablespoons olive oil
- 1 tablespoon cilantro, minced
- 2 sweet corn ears, without husks
- ¼ teaspoon cayenne pepper
- 2 poblano pepper
- ½ cup milk
- 1 teaspoon ground cumin
- 1 tablespoon lime juice
- 1 jalapeno pepper, seeded and minced
- ½ cup sour cream
- 1 and ½ teaspoon garlic salt

Directions:

1. Drain the potatoes and rub them well with oil
2. Preheat Ninja Foodi by pressing the "GRILL" option and setting it to "MED" and timer to 10 minutes
3. Let it preheat until you hear a beep
4. Arrange your prepared poblano pepper over the grill grate, lock lid and cook for 5 minutes
5. Flip the peppers and cook for 5 minutes more
6. Grill the remaining vegetables in the same manner with 7 minutes each side for the potatoes and corn
7. Take a bowl and whisk in remaining ingredients to prepare the vinaigrette
8. Peel the grilled corn and chop
9. Divide corn ears into small pieces and cut your potatoes
10. Serve the grilled veggies with the vinaigrette topping
11. Enjoy!

Nutrition:

Calories: 344, Fat: 5 g, Saturated Fat: 1 g, Carbohydrates: 51 g, Fiber: 3 g, Sodium: 600 mg, Protein: 5 g

Epic Asparagus

Prep time: 5 - 10 minutes

Cooking time: 15 minutes

Servings:

Ingredients:

- ½ teaspoon pepper
- 1 teaspoon salt
- 2 tablespoons olive oil
- ¼ cup honey
- 4 tablespoons tarragon, minced
- 2 pounds asparagus, trimmed

Directions:

1. Take a bowl and add asparagus, honey, oil, pepper, and tarragon
2. Toss well to mix everything
3. Pre-heat your Ninja Foodi Grill to MED and set the timer to 8 minutes
4. Once you hear the beep, transfer asparagus to grill grate and lock lid, cook for 4 minutes
5. Flip and cook for 4 minutes more
6. Serve and enjoy!

Nutrition:

Calories: 240, Fat: 15 g, Saturated Fat: 3 g, Carbohydrates: 31 g, Fiber: 1 g, Sodium: 103 mg, Protein: 7 g

Delicious Broccoli and Arugula

Prep Time: 10 minutes

Cooking Time: 12 minutes

Servings: 4

Ingredients:

- Pepper as needed
- ½ teaspoon salt
- Red pepper flakes
- 2 tablespoons extra virgin olive oil
- 1 tablespoon canola oil
- ½ red onion, sliced
- 1 garlic cloves, minced
- 1 teaspoon Dijon mustard
- 1 teaspoon honey
- 1 tablespoon lemon juice
- 2 tablespoons parmesan cheese, grated
- 4 cups arugula, torn
- 2 heads broccoli, trimmed

Directions:

1. Pre-heat your Ninja Foodi Grill to MAX and set the timer to 12 minutes
2. Take a large-sized bowl and add broccoli, sliced onion, and canola oil, toss the mixture well until coated
3. Once you hear the beep, it is pre-heated
4. Arrange your vegetables over the grill grate, let them grill for 8-12 minutes
5. Take a medium-sized bowl and whisk in lemon juice, olive oil, mustard, honey, garlic, red pepper flakes, pepper, and salt
6. Once done, add the prepared veggies and arugula in a bowl
7. Drizzle the prepared vinaigrette on top, sprinkle a bit of parmesan
8. Stir and mix
9. Enjoy!

Nutrition:

Calories: 168, Fat: 12 g, Saturated Fat: 3 g, Carbohydrates: 13 g, Fiber: 1 g, Sodium: 392 mg, Protein: 6 g

Exciting Granola Muffins

Prep time: 10 minutes

Cooking time:15-20 minutes

Servings: 4

Ingredients:

- 1 tablespoon coriander
- A handful of thyme diced
- ¼ cup of coconut milk
- 3 handful of cooked vegetables of your choice
- 3 ounce plain granola
- Salt and pepper to taste

Directions:

1. Press the "AIR CRISP" option and set this in "352 Degrees F" to pre-heat Ninja Foodi with a 20 minutes timer

2. In a mixing bowl, take cooked vegetables

3. Then take your immersion blender and whiz granola until you have a breadcrumb-like texture

4. Put coconut milk to the granola and also veggies

5. Then mix them well and make muffin/ball shapes of that mixture

6. Onward, shift them to pre-heated Ninja Foodi Grill and let it cook for 20 minutes

7. When it is done, serve, and enjoy!

Nutrition:

Calories: 265, Fat: 12 g, Carbohydrates: 34 g, Protein: 5 g, Sodium: 310 mg, Fiber: 6 g, Saturated Fat: 4 g

Corn and Mayo

Prep Time: 5-10 minutes

Cooking Time: 12 minutes

Servings: 4

Ingredients:

- 2 tablespoons plain yogurt
- 4 ears corn, husked
- ½ teaspoon chili powder
- 2 tablespoon mayonnaise
- 4 tablespoons finely shredded parmesan, cheese
- 1 lime, quartered

Directions:

1. Take a mixing bowl and add yogurt, mayonnaise, chili powder, mix well

2. Take your Ninja Foodi Grill and press "GRILL" and set to "LOW" mode, set the timer to 12 minutes

3. Let it preheat

4. Once you hear a beep, arrange corn over the grill grate

5. Lock lid and cook for 6 minutes, flip and cook for 6 minutes more

6. Serve with prepared sauce, add cheese on top

7. Serve with warm lime wedges, enjoy!

Nutrition:

Calories: 286, Fat: 4 g, Saturated Fat: 1 g, Carbohydrates: 22 g, Fiber: 6 g, Sodium: 542 mg, Protein: 4 g

Fruit Packed Lime Salad

Prep Time: 5-10 minutes
Cooking Time: 4 minutes
Servings: 4
Ingredients:

- ½ pound strawberries washed, hulled and halved
- 1 can (9 ounces) pineapple chunks, drained, juice reserved
- 2 peaches, pitted and sliced
- 6 tablespoons honey, divided
- 1 tablespoon freshly squeezed lime juice

Directions:

1. Take a large bowl and add strawberries, pineapple, peaches, and 3 tablespoons, honey, toss well
2. Preheat Ninja Foodi by pressing the "GRILL" option and setting it to "MAX" and timer to 4 minutes
3. Let it preheat until you hear a beep
4. Transfer fruits to Grill Grate, lock lid and cook for 4 minutes
5. Take a small-sized bowl and add remaining 3 tablespoons of honey, lime juice, 1 tablespoon reserved pineapple juice
6. Once cooking is done, place fruits in a large-sized bowl and toss with honey mixture, serve and enjoy!

Nutrition:
Calories: 178, Fat: 1 g, Saturated Fat: 0 g, Carbohydrates:47 g, Fiber: 3 g, Sodium: 3 mg, Protein: 2 g

Chapter 7: Fish and Seafood

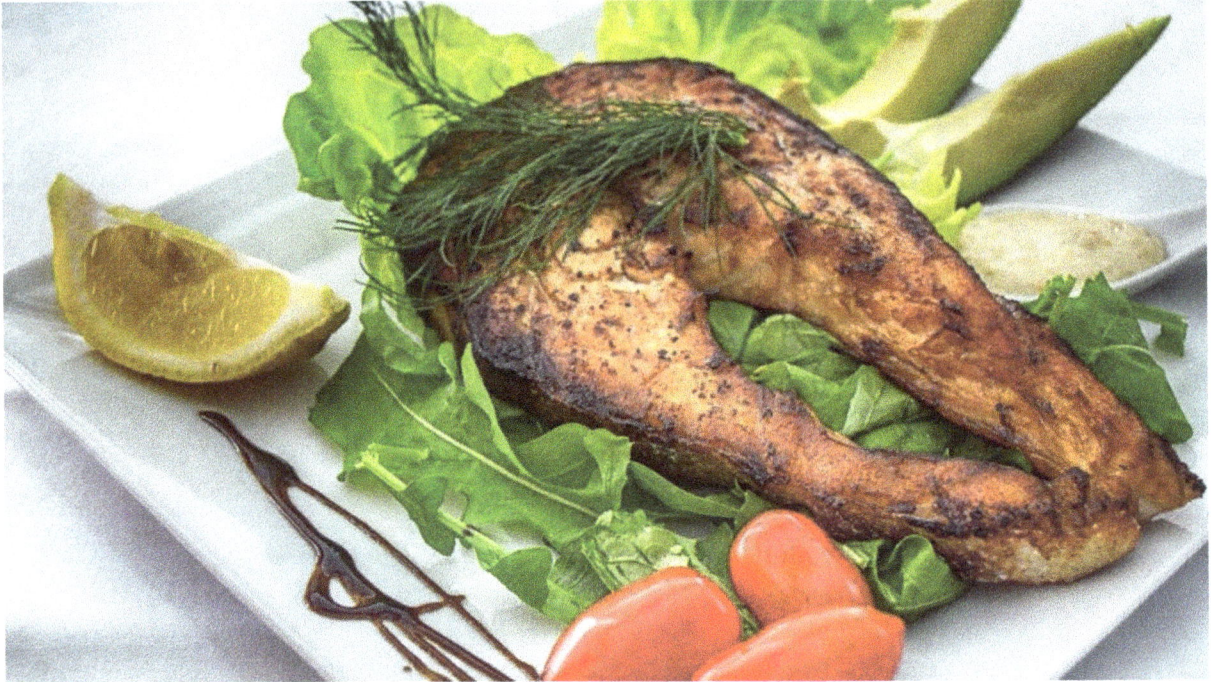

11.

Spanish Shrimp

Prep Time: 5 minutes

Cooking Time: 3 minutes

Serves: 4

Ingredients:

- 2 garlic cloves, minced
- 1½ pounds shelled and deveined medium shrimp
- ½ cup olive oil
- ½ teaspoon salt
- ½ teaspoon red pepper flakes
- 1 lemon, cut into wedges

Directions:

1. Rinse the shrimp and pat dry with paper towels. Combine the shrimp, olive oil, garlic, salt, and red pepper flakes in a medium bowl. Toss gently to combine. Cover with plastic wrap and then refrigerate for at least 30 minutes or up to 2 hours.

2. Insert the Grill Grate and close the hood. Select GRILL, set temperature to HIGH, and set time to 8 minutes. Select START/STOP to begin preheating.

3. Grill the shrimp for about 3 minutes, until they are opaque and firm to the touch. Serve the shrimp immediately in 4 small bowls with the lemon wedges.

Nutrition:

Calories 305, Fat 17 g, Protein 35 g

Mustard Crispy Cod

Prep Time: 5-10 minutes

Cooking Time: 10 minutes

Servings: 3

Ingredients:

- 1 large whole egg
- 1 teaspoon Dijon mustard
- ½ cup breadcrumbs
- 1-pound cod filets
- ¼ cup all-purpose flour
- 1 tablespoon dried parsley
- 1 teaspoon paprika
- ½ teaspoon pepper

Directions:

1. Take fish filets and cut them into 1-inch wide strips

2. Take a blending bowl and speed in eggs, include mustard and consolidate well

3. Include flour in another bowl

4. Take another bowl and include breadcrumbs, dried parsley, paprika, dark pepper and join well

5. Coat strips with flour, at that point cover with egg blend, and cover with scraps finally

6. Pre-heat Ninja Foodi by squeezing the "AIR CRISP" alternative and setting it to "390 Degrees F" and clock to 10 minutes

7. Let it pre-heat until you hear a beep

8. Arrange strips directly inside basket, lock lid and cook until the timer runs out

9. Serve and enjoy!

Nutrition:

Calories: 200, Fat: 4 g, Saturated Fat: 1 g, Carbohydrates: 17 g, Fiber: 1 g, Sodium: 214 mg, Protein: 24 g

Mesmerizing Parmesan Fish

Prep Time: 5-10 minutes

Cooking Time: 13 minutes

Serves: 3

Ingredients:

- ¼ teaspoon salt
- ¾ cup breadcrumbs
- ¼ cup parmesan cheese, grated
- 1-pound haddock fillets
- ¼ teaspoon ground dried thyme
- ¼ cup butter, melted
- ¾ cup milk

Directions:

1. Coat fish fillets in milk, season with salt and keep it on the side

2. Take a mixing bowl and add breadcrumbs, parmesan, cheese, thyme and combine well

3. Coat fillets in bread crumb mixture

4. Pre-heat Ninja Foodi by pressing the "BAKE" option and setting it to "325 Degrees F" and timer to 13 minutes

5. Let it pre-heat until you hear a beep

6. Arrange fish fillets directly over Grill Grate, lock lid and cook for 8 minutes, flip and cook for the remaining time

7. Serve and enjoy!

Nutrition:

Calories: 450, Fat: 27 g, Saturated Fat: 12 g, Carbohydrates: 16 g, Fiber: 3 g, Sodium: 1056 mg, Protein: 44 g

Lemon Garlic Shrimp

Prep Time: 40 minutes

Serves: 4

Ingredients:

- 1 lb. shrimp, peeled and deveined

- 4 cloves garlic, minced

- 1 tablespoon lemon juice

- 1 tablespoon olive oil

- Salt to taste

Directions:

1. Mix the olive oil, salt, lemon juice, and garlic. Toss shrimp in the mixture.

2. Marinate for 15 minutes. Place the shrimp in the Ninja Foodi basket.

3. Seal the crisping lid. Select the crisp air setting.

4. Cook at 350 degrees for 8 minutes. Flip and cook for 2 more minutes.

Serving Suggestion: Sprinkle chopped parsley on top.

Tip: Add crushed red pepper flakes if you like it spicy.

Nutrition:

Calories 170, Total Fat 5.5g, Saturated Fat 1.1g, Cholesterol 239mg, Sodium 317mg, Total Carbohydrate 2.8g, Dietary Fiber 0.1g, Total Sugars 0.1g, Protein 26.1g, Potassium 209mg

Tuna Patties

Serves: 2

Prep Time: 30 minutes

Ingredients:

- 2 cans tuna flakes
- 1 tablespoon mayo
- 1 teaspoon garlic powder
- 1/2 teaspoon onion powder
- 1/2 tablespoon almond flour
- 1 teaspoon dried dill
- Salt and pepper to taste
- 1 tablespoon lemon juice

Directions:

1. Mix all the ingredients in a bowl. Form patties. Set the tuna patties on the Ninja Foodi basket. Seal the crisping lid. Set it to air crisp.
2. Cook at 400 degrees for 10 minutes. Flip and cook for 5 more minutes.

Serving Suggestion: Serve with a fresh green salad.

Tip: Add more flour if too wet.

Nutrition:

Calories 141, Total Fat 6.4g, Saturated Fat 0.7g, Cholesterol 17mg, Sodium 148mg, Total Carbohydrate 5.2g, Dietary Fiber 1g, Total Sugars 1.2g, Protein 17g, Potassium 48mg

Roast BBQ Shrimp

Prep Time: 5-10 minutes

Cooking Time: 7 minutes

Servings: 2

Ingredients:

- 3 tablespoons chipotle in adobo sauce, minced
- ¼ teaspoon salt

- ¼ cup BBQ sauce

- ½ orange, juiced

- ½ pound large shrimps

Directions:

1. Take a mixing bowl and add all ingredients, mix well

2. Keep it on the side

3. Pre-heat Ninja Foodi by pressing the "ROAST" option and setting it to "400 Degrees F" and timer to 7 minutes

4. Let it pre-heat until you hear a beep

5. Arrange shrimps over Grill Grate and lock lid, cook until the timer runs out

6. Serve and enjoy!

Nutrition:

Calories: 173, Fat: 2 g, Saturated Fat: 0.5 g, Carbohydrates: 21 g, Fiber: 2 g, Sodium: 1143 mg, Protein: 17 g

Crispy Crabby Patties

Prep Time: 5-10 minutes

Cooking Time: 10 minutes

Servings: 4

Ingredients:

- 1 shallot, minced

- ¼ cup mayonnaise, low carb

- 12 ounces lump crabmeat

- ¼ cup parsley, minced

- 2 tablespoons Dijon mustard

- 2 tablespoons almond flour

- 1 lemon, zest

- 1 egg, beaten

- Pepper and salt as needed

Directions:

1. Take a mixing bowl and add all ingredients, mix well and prepare 4 meat from the mixture

2. Pre-heat Ninja Foodi by squeezing the "AIR CRISP" choice and setting it to "375 Degrees F" and timer to 10 minutes

3. Let it pre-heat until you hear a beep

4. Transfer patties to cooking basket and let them cook for 5 minutes, flip and cook for 5 minutes more

5. Serve and enjoy once done!

Nutrition:

Calories: 177, Fat: 13 g, Saturated Fat: 2 g, Carbohydrates: 2.5 g, Fiber: 0 g, Sodium: 358 mg, Protein: 11 g

Tuna Patties

Prep Time: 30 minutes

Serves: 2

Ingredients:

- 1 teaspoon garlic powder
- 1 tablespoon lemon juice
- 2 cans tuna flakes
- 1 tablespoon mayo
- 1/2 tablespoon almond flour
- 1/2 teaspoon onion powder
- 1 teaspoon dried dill
- Salt and pepper to taste

Directions:

1. Mix all the ingredients in a bowl. Form patties. Set the tuna patties on the Ninja Foodi basket. Seal the crisping lid. Set it to air crisp.

2. Cook at 400 degrees for 10 minutes. Flip and cook for 5 more minutes.

Serving Suggestion: Serve with a fresh green salad.

Tip: Add more flour if too wet.

Nutrition:

Calories 141, Total Fat 6.4g, Saturated Fat 0.7g, Cholesterol 17mg, Sodium 148mg, Total Carbohydrate 5.2g, Dietary Fiber 1g, Total Sugars 1.2g, Protein 17g, Potassium 48mg

Salt and Pepper Shrimp

Prep Time: 20 minutes

Serves: 4

Ingredients:

- 2 teaspoons peppercorns
- 1 lb. shrimp
- 1 teaspoons sugar
- 3 tablespoons rice flour
- 1 teaspoon salt
- 2 tablespoons oil

Directions:

1. Set the Ninja Foodi Grill to Roast the peppercorns for 1 minute. Let them cool.
2. Crush the peppercorns and add the salt and sugar.
3. Coat the shrimp with this mixture and then with flour.
4. Sprinkle oil on the Ninja Foodi basket. Place the shrimp on top.
5. Cook at 350 degrees for 10 minutes, flipping halfway through.

Serving Suggestion: Serve with fresh salad.

Tip: Add more peppercorns if you like it spicier.

Nutrition:

Calories 228, Total Fat 8.9g, Saturated Fat 1.5g, Cholesterol 239mg, Sodium 859mg, Total Carbohydrate 9.3g, Dietary Fiber 0.5g, Total Sugars 1g, Protein 26.4g, Potassium 211mg

Spicy Grilled Shrimps

Prep Time: 5-10 minutes

Cooking Time: 6 minutes

Servings: 4

Ingredients:

- 1 teaspoon garlic salt
- ½ teaspoon black pepper
- 1 tablespoon paprika
- 1 tablespoon garlic powder
- 2 tablespoons olive oil
- 1-pound jumbo shrimps, peeled and deveined
- 2 tablespoons brown sugar

Directions:

1. Take a mixing bowl and add listed ingredients to mix well
2. Let it chill and marinate for 30-60 minutes
3. Pre-heat Ninja Foodi by pressing the "GRILL" option and setting it to "MED" and timer to 6 minutes
4. Let it pre-heat until you hear a beep
5. Arrange prepared shrimps over grill grate, lock lid and cook for 3 minutes, flip and cook for 3 minutes more
6. Serve and enjoy!

Nutrition:

Calories: 370, Fat: 27 g, Saturated Fat: 3 g, Carbohydrates: 23 g, Fiber: 8 g, Sodium: 182 mg, Protein: 6 g

Buttery Spiced Grilled Salmon

Prep Time: 5-10 minutes

Cooking Time: 10 minutes

Servings: 4

Ingredients:

- 2 teaspoons cayenne pepper
- 2 pounds salmon fillets

- 2 teaspoon salt
- 6 tablespoons butter, melted
- 1 and ¼ teaspoon onion salt
- 2 tablespoons lemon pepper
- 1 teaspoon white pepper, ground
- 1 teaspoon black pepper, ground
- 1 teaspoon dry basil
- 1 teaspoon ancho chili powder
- 1 teaspoon dry oregano
- Lemon wedges and dill sprigs

Directions:

1. Season salmon fillets with butter, take a mixing bowl and add listed ingredients
2. Coat salmon fillets with the mixture
3. Pre-heat Ninja Foodi by pressing the "GRILL" option and setting it to "MED" and timer to 10 minutes
4. Let it pre-heat until you hear a beep
5. Arrange prepared fillets over grill grate, let them cook for 5 minutes, flip and cook for 5 minutes more
6. Serve and enjoy!

Nutrition:

Calories: 300, Fat: 8 g, Saturated Fat: 2 g, Carbohydrates: 17 g, Fiber: 1 g, Sodium: 342 mg, Protein: 26 g

Teriyaki Coho Glazed Salmon

Prep Time: 10 minutes

Cooking Time: 25 minutes

Serves: 4

Ingredients:

- 1-2 coho salmon filets
- 1 tablespoon honey

- 1 and ½ tablespoons ginger roots, minced
- 2 tablespoons cornstarch
- 1 cup of water
- ¼ cup of soy sauce
- ¼ cup brown sugar
- ½ teaspoon white pepper
- ¼ cup of cold water

Directions:

1. Insert the grill grate and close the hood
2. Pre-heat Ninja Foodi by pressing the "GRILL" option and setting it to "HIGH" for 15 minutes
3. Take a medium saucepan over medium heat, combine sauce ingredients (except salmon, cornstarch and cold water) and bring to a low boil
4. Then add cornstarch and water in another bowl, whisk cornstarch mixture slowly into sauce until it thickens
5. Add one chunk of pecan wood to the hot coal of your grill
6. Brush sauce onto the salmon filet
7. Place on the grill grate, then close the hood
8. Cook for 15 minutes
9. Brush the salmon with another coat of sauce
10. Close the lid and cook for 10 minutes more
11. Serve and enjoy!

Nutrition:

Calories: 163, Fat: 0 g, Saturated Fat: 0 g, Carbohydrates: 15 g, Fiber: 3 g, Sodium: 456 mg, Protein: 0 g

Simple Grilled Swordfish

Prep Time: 5 minutes

Cooking Time: 4 minutes

Serves: 4

Ingredients:

- 4 (6-ounce swordfish steaks, about I inch thick
- Juice of ½ lemon
- ½ teaspoon dried oregano
- ¼ cup olive oil

Directions:

1. Rinse the fish and pat dry with paper towels.
2. Combine the olive oil, lemon juice, and oregano in a shallow baking dish large enough to fit all the swordfish steaks. Add the swordfish steaks and marinate for about 15 minutes. Turn the steaks and marinate for another 15 minutes.
3. Insert the Grill Grate and close the hood. Select GRILL, set temperature to HIGH, and set time to 8 minutes. Select START/STOP to begin preheating.
4. Sprinkle the swordfish steaks with the salt and pepper—grill for about 4 minutes. To test for doneness, prod an edge of the swordfish with a fork. The fish should flake easily. Serve immediately.

Nutrition:

Calories 327, Fat 21 g, Protein 34 g

Coconut Shrimp

Prep Time: 20 minutes

Serves: 4

Ingredients:

- 1/2 cup all-purpose flour
- 1/3 cup panko bread crumbs
- 2/3 cup unsweetened coconut flakes
- 1/4 cup honey
- 1-1/2 teaspoons black pepper
- Cooking spray
- 2 eggs
- 12 oz. shrimp, peeled and deveined

- Salt and pepper to taste
- 1/4 cup lime juice

Directions:

1. Mix the flour and black pepper in a bowl. In another bowl, beat the egg.
2. In the third bowl, mix the bread crumbs and coconut flakes.
3. Dip each of the shrimp in the first, second, and third bowls.
4. Place in the Ninja Foodi basket. Set it to air crisp. Cover the crisping lid.
5. Cook at 400 degrees F for 8 minutes, turning halfway through.
6. Season with the salt and pepper.
7. Mix the remaining ingredients and serve with the shrimp.

Serving Suggestion: Garnish with fresh cilantro.

Tip: Keep the tails of the shrimp.

Nutrition:

Calories 293, Total Fat 4.4g, Saturated Fat 1.3g, Cholesterol 261mg, Sodium 306mg, Total Carbohydrate 37.8g, Dietary Fiber 1.1g, Total Sugars 18.2g, Protein 25.1g, Potassium 229mg

-

Chapter 8: Desserts, Bread & Rolls

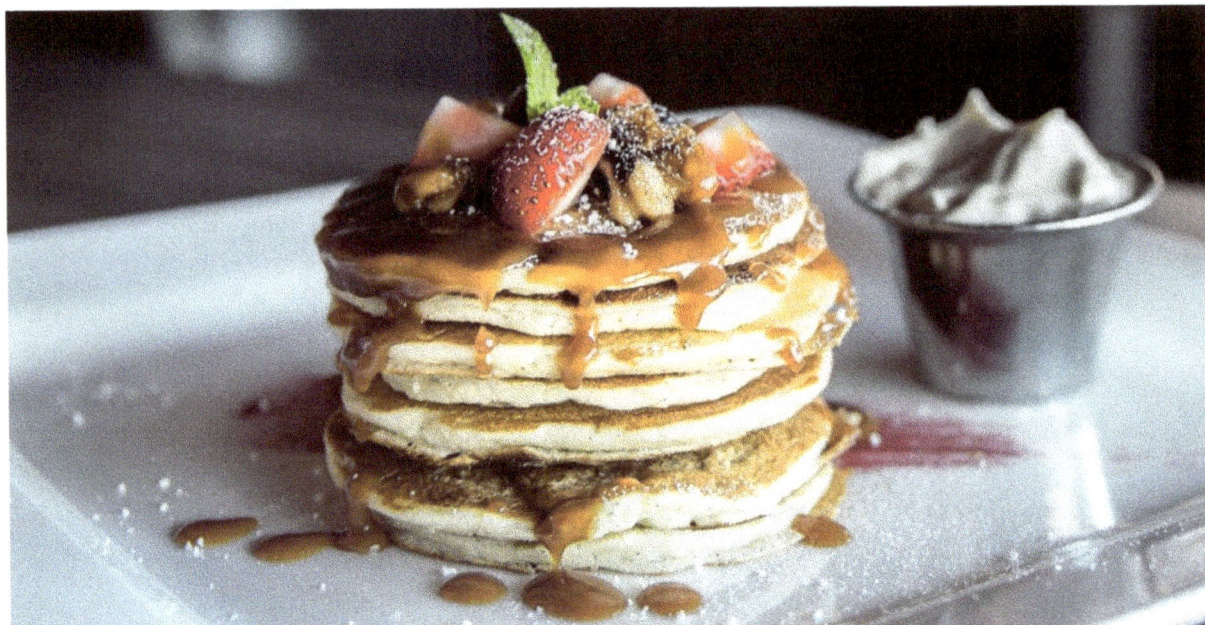

12.

A Fruit Salad to Die For

- Prep Time: 5-10 minutes

Cooking Time: 4 minutes

Servings: 4

Ingredients:

- 2 peaches, pitted and sliced
- 1 can (9 ounces) pineapple chunks, drained, juice reserved
- ½ pound strawberries washed, hulled and halved
- 1 tablespoon freshly squeezed lime juice
- 6 tablespoons honey, divided

Directions:

1. Add pineapple, peaches, strawberries, and ½ of honey, toss well
2. Pre-heat your Ninja Foodi by pressing the "GRILL" option and setting it to "MAX."
3. Set the timer to 4 minutes
4. Allow it to pre-heat until it beeps

5. Transfer fruits to Grill Grate and close the lid

6. Cook for 4 minutes

7. Add remaining 3 tablespoons of honey, lime juice, 1 tablespoon reserved pineapple juice into a small-sized bowl

8. Once cooked, place fruits in a large-sized bowl and toss with honey mixture

9. Serve and enjoy!

Nutrition:
Calories: 178, Fat: 1 g, Saturated Fat: 0 g, Carbohydrates:47 g, Fiber: 3 g, Sodium: 3 mg, Protein: 2 g

11.

French Toast Bites

• Prep Time: 5 minutes
Cooking Time: 15 minutes
Serving: 8
Ingredients:

- Almond milk

- Cinnamon

- Sweetener

- 3 eggs

- 4 pieces wheat bread

Directions:

1. Insert the Crisper Basket, and close the hood. Select AIR CRISP, set the temperature to 360°F, and set the time to 15 minutes. Select START/STOP to begin preheating.

2. Whisk eggs and thin out with almond milk.

3. Mix 1/3 cup of sweetener with lots of cinnamon.

4. Tear bread in half, ball up pieces and press together to form a ball.

5. Soak bread balls in egg and then roll into cinnamon sugar, making sure to thoroughly coat.

6. Air frying. Place coated bread balls into the air fryer and bake 15 minutes.

Nutrition:
Calories 300, Fat 10 g, Protein 2 g, Sugar 4 g

12.

Lovely Rum Sundae

- Prep Time: 10 minutes

Cooking Time: 8 minutes

Servings: 4

Ingredients:

- Vanilla ice cream for serving
- 1 pineapple, cored and sliced
- 1 teaspoon cinnamon, ground
- ½ cup brown sugar, packed
- ½ cup dark rum

Directions:

1. Take a large deep bowl and add sugar, cinnamon, and rum
2. Add the pineapple in the layer, dredge them properly and make sure that they are coated well
3. Pre-heat your Foodi in "GRILL" mode with "MAX" settings, setting the timer to 8 minutes
4. Once you hear the beep, strain any additional rum from the pineapple slices and transfer them to the grill rate of your appliance
5. Press them down and grill for 6-8 minutes. Make sure to not overcrowd the grill grate, Cook in batches if needed
6. Top each of the ring with a scoop of your favorite ice cream, sprinkle a bit of cinnamon on top
7. Enjoy!

Nutrition:

Calories: 240, Fat: 4 g, Saturated Fat: 1 g, Carbohydrates: 43 g, Fiber: 8 g, Sodium: 85 mg, Protein: 2 g

13.

Fiery Cajun Eggplant Dish

- Prep Time: 5-10 minutes

Cooking Time: 12 minutes

Servings: 4

Ingredients:

- 2 tablespoons lime juice

- 3 teaspoons Cajun seasoning
- 2 small eggplants, cut into slices
- ¼ cup olive oil

Directions:

1. Coat eggplant slices with oil, lemon juice, and Cajun seasoning
2. Take your Ninja Foodi Grill and press "GRILL" and set to "MED" mode, set the timer to 10 minutes
3. Let it preheat
4. Arrange eggplants over grill grate, lock lid and cook for 5 minutes
5. Flip and cook for 5 minutes more
6. Serve and enjoy!

Nutrition:
Calories: 362, Fat: 11 g, Saturated Fat: 3 g, Carbohydrates: 16 g, Fiber: 1 g, Sodium: 694 mg, Protein: 8 g

14.

Granola Flavored Healthy Muffin

- Prep Time: 10 minutes

Cooking Time: 15-20 minutes

Servings: 4

Ingredients:

- 3 ounces plain granola
- 3 handful of cooked vegetables of your choice
- ¼ cup of coconut milk
- A handful of thyme diced
- 1 tablespoon coriander
- Salt and pepper to taste

Directions:

1. Preheat Ninja Foodi by pressing the "AIR CRISP" option and setting it to "352 Degrees F" and timer to 20 minutes
2. Take a mixing bowl and add cooked vegetables
3. Take an immersion blender and whiz granola until you have a breadcrumb-like texture

4. Add coconut milk to the granola and add veggies

5. Mix well into muffin/ball shapes

6. Transfer them to preheated Ninja Foodi Grill and cook for 20 minutes

7. Serve and enjoy once done!

Nutrition:
Calories: 140, Fat: 10 g, Saturated Fat: 3 g, Carbohydrates: 14 g, Fiber: 4 g, Sodium: 215 mg, Protein: 2 g

15.

Cinnamon Sugar Roasted Chickpeas

- Prep Time: 5 minutes

Cooking Time: 10 minutes
Serving: 2
Ingredients:

- 1 tbsp. sweetener

- 1 tbsp. cinnamon

- 1 C. chickpeas

Directions:

1. Insert the Crisper Basket, and close the hood. Select AIR CRISP, set the temperature to 390°F, and set the time to 10 minutes. Select START/STOP to begin preheating.

2. Rinse and drain chickpeas.

3. Mix all ingredients together and add to Grill.

4. Air frying. Cook 10 minutes.

Nutrition:
Calories 115, Fat 20 g, Protein 18 g, Sugar 7 g

16.

Marshmallow Banana Boat

- Prep Time: 19 minutes

Cooking Time: 6 minutes
Servings: 4
Ingredients:

- ½ cup peanut butter chips

- 1/3 cup chocolate chips

- 1 cup mini marshmallow
- 4 ripe bananas

Directions:

1. Take the banana and slice them gently, keeping the peel
2. Make sure to not cut it all the way through
3. Use your hands to carefully peel the banana skin like a book, revealing the banana flesh
4. Divide your marshmallow, peanut butter, chocolate chips among the prepared bananas, stuff them well
5. Preheat your Grill in "MEDIUM" mode, with the timer set to 6 minutes
6. Once you hear a beep, transfer your prepared bananas to grill grate, cook for 4-6 minutes until the chocolate melts well
7. Serve and enjoy!

Nutrition:
Calories: 505, Fat: 18 g, Saturated Fat: 4 g, Carbohydrates: 82 g, Fiber: 6 g, Sodium: 166 mg, Protein: 10 g

17.

Smoked Apple Crumble

- Prep Time: 5 minutes

Cooking Time: 45 minutes
Serving: 4
Ingredients:
Filling

- 4–5 large Honeycrisp apples, peeled and sliced
- juice from ½ lemon
- 2 Tbsp. flour
- ⅓ cup sugar
- 1 Tbsp. ground cinnamon
- 1 tsp. ground nutmeg

Topping

- 1 cup brown sugar
- ½ cup flour

- ½ cup oatmeal
- ½ cup caramel baking chips
- ¼ cup candied pecans
- 1 Tbsp. ground cinnamon
- 1 tsp. baking powder
- ½ tsp. salt
- ½ cup salted butter, cold and cut into small chunks

Directions:

1. Insert the Grill Grate and close the hood. Select GRILL, set temperature to HIGH, and set time to 40 minutes. Select START/STOP to begin preheating.

2. Place apples in a large mixing bowl and toss with lemon juice. Then add in flour, sugar, cinnamon, and nutmeg, and mix thoroughly.

3. Pour apples into a greased cast-iron pan. Set mixture aside.

4. Using the now-empty mixing bowl, combine brown sugar, flour, oatmeal, caramel chips, pecans, cinnamon, baking powder, and salt for the topping.

5. Using a pastry blender or large fork, cut the cold butter into the topping mix.

6. Cover apples with topping mixture.

7. Add one or two pecan wood chunks to the hot coals. Place apple crumble over the Roasting Rack.

8. Close the hood and bake until apples start to bubble and topping begins to brown (about 45 minutes).

9. Remove from grill and serve warm with French vanilla ice cream.

18.

Sweet Cream Cheese Wontons

- Prep Time: 5 minutes

Cooking Time: 5 minutes
Serving: 16
Ingredients:

- 1 egg mixed with a bit of water
- Wonton wrappers
- ½ C. powdered erythritol

- 8 ounces softened cream cheese
- Olive oil

Directions:

1. Mix sweetener and cream cheese together.
2. Lay out 4 wontons at a time and cover with a dish towel to prevent drying out.
3. Place ½ of a teaspoon of cream cheese mixture into each wrapper.
4. Dip finger into egg/water mixture and fold diagonally to form a triangle. Seal edges well.
5. Repeat with remaining ingredients.
6. Insert the Crisper Basket, and close the hood. Select AIR CRISP, set the temperature to 400°F, and set the time to 5 minutes. Select START/STOP to begin preheating.
7. Air frying. Place filled wontons into the Grill and cook 5 minutes at 400 degrees, shaking halfway through cooking.

Nutrition:
Calories 303, Fat 3 g, Protein 1 g, Sugar 4 g

19.

Tuna Stuffed Potatoes

- Prep Time: 5 minutes

Cooking Time: 30 minutes
Serving: 4

Ingredients:

- 4 starchy potatoes
- ½ tablespoon olive oil
- 1 (6-ounce can tuna, drained
- 2 tablespoons plain Greek yogurt
- 1 teaspoon red chili powder
- Salt and freshly ground black pepper, to taste
- 1 scallion, chopped and divided
- 1 tablespoon capers

Directions:

1. In a large bowl of water, soak the potatoes for about 30 minutes. Drain well and pat dry with a paper towel.

2. Insert the Crisper Basket, and close the hood. Select AIR CRISP, set the temperature to 355°F, and set the time to 30 minutes. Select START/STOP to begin preheating and place the potatoes in the crisper basket.

3. Air Frying.

4. Cook for about 30 minutes.

5. Meanwhile, in a bowl, add tuna, yogurt, red chili powder, salt, black pepper, and half of the scallion, and with a potato masher, mash the mixture thoroughly.

6. Remove the potatoes from the air fryer and place it onto a smooth surface.

7. Carefully cut each potato from the top side lengthwise.

8. With your fingers, press the open side of potato halves slightly. Stuff the available potato portion with tuna mixture evenly.

9. Sprinkle with the capers and remaining scallion. Serve immediately.

20.

Cinnamon Fried Bananas

- Prep Time: 5 minutes

Cooking Time: 10 minutes
Serving: 2-3
Ingredients:

- 1 C. panko breadcrumbs
- 3 tbsp. cinnamon
- ½ C. almond flour
- 3 egg whites
- 8 ripe bananas
- 3 tbsp. vegan coconut oil

Directions:

1. Heat coconut oil and add breadcrumbs. Mix around 2-3 minutes until golden. Pour into bowl.

2. Peel and cut bananas in half. Roll each bananas half into flour, eggs, and crumb mixture.

3. AIR CRISP. Place into the Ninja Foodi Grill. Cook 10 minutes at 280 degrees.

4. A great addition to a healthy banana split!

Nutrition:

Calories 215, Fat 11 g, Protein 5 g, Sugar 5 g

21.

Bruschetta Portobello Mushrooms

- Prep Time: 10 minutes

Cooking Time: 8 minutes

Serving: 6

Ingredients:

- 2 cups cherry tomatoes, cut in half

- 3 tablespoons red onion, diced

- 3 tablespoons fresh basil shredded

- Salt and black pepper to taste

- 4 tablespoons butter

- 1 teaspoon dried oregano

- 6 large Portobello Mushrooms, caps only, washed and dried

For Balsamic glaze:

- 2 teaspoons brown sugar

- 1/4 cup balsamic vinegar

Directions:

1. Start by preparing the balsamic glaze and take all its ingredients in a saucepan.

2. Stir cook this mixture for 8 minutes on medium heat then remove from the heat.

3. Take the mushrooms and brush them with the prepared glaze.

4. Stuff the remaining ingredients into the mushrooms.

5. Prepare and preheat the Ninja Foodi Grill in the medium-temperature setting.

6. Once it is preheated, open the lid and place the stuffed mushrooms in the grill with their cap side down.

7. Cover the Ninja Foodi Grill's lid and let it grill on the "Grilling Mode" for 8 minutes.

8. Serve.

Nutrition:

Calories 331, Total Fat 2.5 g, Saturated Fat 0.5 g, Cholesterol 35 mg, Sodium 595 mg, Total Carbs 69 g, Fiber 12.2 g, Sugar 12.5 g, Protein 8.7g

Marshmallow Banana Boat

- Prep Time: 19 minutes

Cooking Time: 6 minutes

Servings: 4

Ingredients:

- 4 ripe bananas
- 1 cup mini marshmallows
- ½ cup of chocolate chips
- ½ cup peanut butter chips

Directions:

1. Slice a banana lengthwise, keeping its peel. Make sure to not cut all the way through
2. Use your hands to open banana peel like a book, revealing the inside of a banana
3. Divide marshmallow, chocolate chips, peanut butter among bananas, stuffing them inside
4. Preheat Ninja Foodi by pressing the "GRILL" option and setting it to "MEDIUM" and timer to 6 minutes
5. let it preheat until you hear a beep
6. Transfer banana to Grill Grate and lock lid, cook for 4-6 minutes until chocolate melts and bananas are toasted
7. Serve and enjoy!

Nutrition:

Calories: 505, Fat: 18 g, Saturated Fat: 13 g, Carbohydrates: 82 g, Fiber: 6 g, Sodium: 103 mg, Protein: 10 g

22.

Baked Apple

- Prep Time: 5 minutes

Cooking Time: 20 minutes

Serving: 4

Ingredients:

- ¼ C. water
- ¼ tsp. nutmeg
- ¼ tsp. cinnamon
- 1 ½ tsp. melted ghee
- 2 tbsp. raisins
- 2 tbsp. chopped walnuts
- 1 medium apple

Directions:

1. Insert the Crisper Basket, and close the hood. Select AIR CRISP, set the temperature to 350°F, and set the time to 20 minutes. Select START/STOP to begin preheating.
2. Slice apple in half and discard some of the flesh from the center.
3. Place into frying pan.
4. Mix remaining ingredients together except water. Spoon mixture to the middle of apple halves.
5. Pour water over filled apples.
6. Air frying. Place pan with apple halves into the air fryer, bake 20 minutes.

Nutrition:

Calories 205, Fat 11 g, Protein 2 g, Sugar 5 g

23.

Rummy Pineapple Sunday

- Prep Time: 10 minutes

Cooking Time: 8 minutes

Servings: 4

Ingredients:

- ½ cup dark rum
- ½ cup packed brown sugar
- 1 teaspoon ground cinnamon, plus more for garnish
- 1 pineapple cored and sliced
- Vanilla ice cream, for serving

Directions:

1. Take a large-sized bowl and add rum, sugar, cinnamon

2. Add pineapple slices, arrange them in the layer. Coat mixture then let them soak for 5 minutes, per side

3. Preheat Ninja Foodi by pressing the "GRILL" option and setting it to "MAX" and timer to 8 minutes

4. let it preheat until you hear a beep

5. Strain extra rum sauce from pineapple

6. Transfer prepared fruit in grill grate in a single layer, press down fruit and lock lid

7. Grill for 6-8 minutes without flipping, work in batches if needed

8. Once done, remove and top each pineapple ring with a scoop of ice cream, sprinkle cinnamon and serve

9. Enjoy!

Nutrition:
Calories: 240, Fat: 4 g, Saturated Fat: 2 g, Carbohydrates: 43 g, Fiber: 3 g, Sodium: 32 mg, Protein: 2 g

24.

Cherry-Choco Bars

- Prep Time: 5 minutes

Cooking Time: 15 minutes
Serving: 8

Ingredients:

- ¼ teaspoon salt

- ½ cup almonds, sliced

- ½ cup chia seeds

- ½ cup dark chocolate, chopped

- ½ cup dried cherries, chopped

- ½ cup prunes, pureed

- ½ cup quinoa, cooked

- ¾ cup almond butter

- 1/3 cup honey

- 2 cups old-fashioned oats

- 2 tablespoon coconut oil

Directions:

1. Insert the Crisper Basket, and close the hood. Select AIR CRISP, set the temperature to 375°F, and set the time to 15 minutes. Select START/STOP to begin preheating.

2. In a mixing bowl, combine the oats, quinoa, chia seeds, almond, cherries, and chocolate.

3. In a saucepan, heat the almond butter, honey, and coconut oil.

4. Pour the butter mixture over the dry mixture. Add salt and prunes.

5. Mix until well combined.

6. Pour over a baking dish that can fit inside the Grill.

7. Air frying. Cook for 15 minutes.

8. Let it cool for an hour before slicing into bars.

Nutrition:

Calories 330, Fat 15 g, Protein 7 g, Sugar 8 g